HIGHWAY HYPODERMICS

On The Road Again

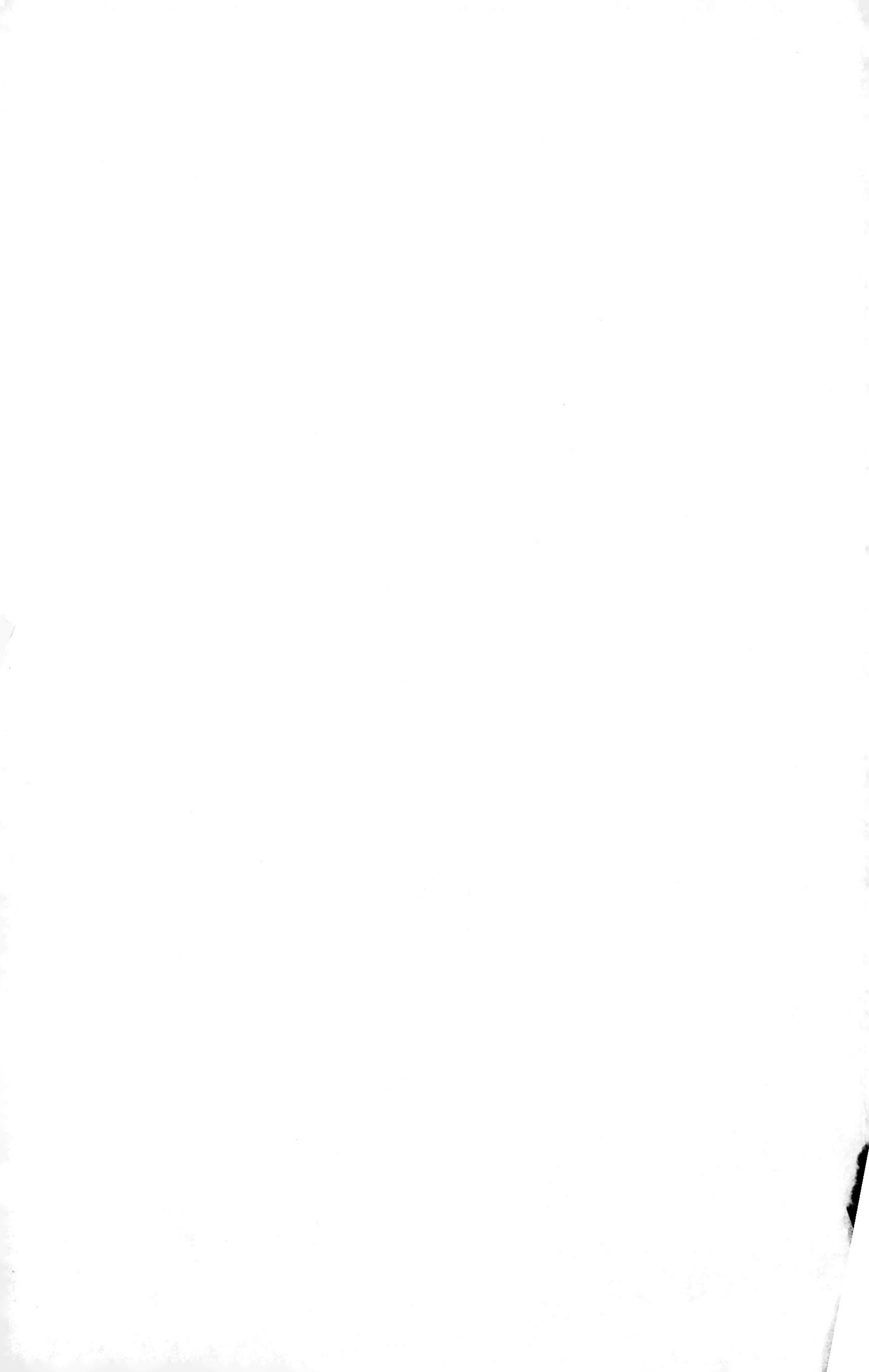

HIGHWAY HYPODERMICS

ON THE ROAD AGAIN

By

Epstein LaRue, RN, BS

Epstein LaRue RnBS

Highway Hypodermics:
On The Road Again

ISBN: 978-1-935188-02-5

Library of Congress Number
LCCN: 2009920457

Edited by Janet Elaine Smith
Interior Design by: Alicia McMullen
Cover Design by Epstein LaRue

Published in 2009 by Star Publish, LLC
Printed in the United States of America

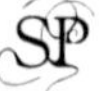

A Star Publish Book
www.starpublishllc.com
Pennsylvania, U.S.A.

Dedicated to:

All the traveling nurses who spend thirteen weeks at a time in a place far away from home—the nurses who are changing healthcare in America one hospital at a time.

All the traveling companies who have supported the Highway Hypodermics book series and website...and especially to those companies who provide great quality service to traveling nurses.

Last, but not least, to my house-husband / home manager / healthcare support team. Thank you for not griping about the dirty dishes and dusty house, taking time to pay the bills, and letting me drag you around the United States all because I love being a traveling nurse and author!

INTERIOR CONTENTS:

Chapter One

The Changing Face of Travel Nursing

Have you seen the price at the gas pumps lately? In July 2006 gas was $2.75 a gallon, and today it's averaging $3.75 a gallon. On my first travel assignment in 2003 I paid rent of $600/month; for the assignment I'm just about to leave on (in 2008), my total housing costs are over $1000/month.

I am starting to see a few changes in the economic status of some travel companies, but surprisingly, most of the companies I have talked to say that there are still plenty of jobs.

It seems that the biggest change is to the nurses themselves with their traveling costs. My question is, if the costs are getting higher for the nurses, who is paying for the extra expenses, or are we just not traveling as often? The hospitals definitely are not...a lot of them struggled to make it before the economical down-slump. I'm really surprised that we haven't seen more of a drop in the amount of travel nursing jobs out there. From my research, it appears that the number of nurses staying at home is directly proportional to the number of jobs that are available.

What nurses have to realize is that there is just so much money that the travel companies are allowed to give out of the bill-rate, and unfortunately, the bill-rates are not going up. I truly believe that most of the companies are doing their best to ease the pain, but the hospitals are not giving out more money to cover some of the additional costs.

What companies have to realize is that it is getting harder and harder to make a living on the road with all the added expenses related to traveling fulltime, especially if you love to make those across-the-country jaunts! Two months ago I came home to Idaho from my assignment in Myrtle Beach, South Carolina, and it cost me $1000.00 for the trip just for the gas. Depending on where your assignment is, that is a paycheck or two just for traveling expenses.

What are the true effects? The hospital's need for traveling nurses will decline as it is related to more traveling nurses staying at home and doing per diem, but for those of us who stay out on the road there will be plenty of jobs left due to less nurses wanting those jobs. I also see that the higher wages that traveling nurses make over the staff nurse is being eaten up in traveling costs. I can definitely see more nurses taking twenty-six week contracts instead of just thirteen-week contracts and traveling closer to home.

It may be a little bumpy on the road and we might even see a washboard effect when the government tries to fix things, but there will always be dedicated traveling nurses and dedicated traveling companies that will carry on until they find the pavement and head down the smooth highway of travel nursing once again.

Through educating yourself with this book and the resources mentioned in this book you can have a very profitable travel nursing career, not only financially but personally, you can bring a wealth of information to other nurses who would like the freedom that travel nursing brings.

My Start as a Traveling Nurse

From the moment I became a nurse in 1992 until I hit the road in 2003, I had always dreamed of being a traveling nurse. It was in a small nursing home in Oklahoma that I met my first travel nurse from South Dakota. The stories that she would tell! They were all full of excitement and it seemed like there was never a dull moment.

It was then that I planned my strategy for becoming a traveling nurse by getting as much experience as I could in all the different areas of nursing. I started working long-term care, then I progressed to medical, surgical, rehab, psych, and eventually into the emergency room.

All this time, I was waiting on my son to graduate from school so we could go on the road, until one day the school counselor told me that he didn't know what he was going to do with my son next year. I looked at my husband, then back at the counselor and told him that I didn't think that he was going to have to worry about my son. I turned in my two-weeks notice at work and we notified the state of Arizona of our intent to home school our child, and off to Phoenix from Lake Havasu City we went.

That was in 2003 and we haven't once looked back. Since then we have been to California, back to Arizona, Oklahoma, Mississippi, Iowa, Florida, Tennessee, Washington (where my son stayed since he turned 18), Oregon, and South Carolina. The first of November my healthcare support assistant (hubby) and I are starting a new assignment in the state of Texas. We have been through earthquakes in California, a gas pipeline crisis in Arizona, missed the tornado in Iowa and Tennessee, and survived one of the worst snow storms of the decade in the Seattle area. I wouldn't trade a minute of it for a staff nurse job! I can't wait to see what Texas will bring!

Anyway, back to 2003. At that time I already had two published novels (*Love At First Type* and *Crazy Thoughts of Passion*), and the minute I started traveling I started gathering information from travel companies and from older travelers. Instead of keeping all of that information to myself I started the website Highway Hypodermics and immediately started putting together *Highway Hypodermics: Your Road to Travel Nursing,* which was published in January 2005.

In Jaunary 2007, Star Publish and I put out the second edition, Highway Hypodermics: Travel Nursing *2007.* In that edition there was a lot of information added about the PBDS test, JCAHO, homeschooling and traveling with family.

Well, it's September 2008 now, and here I am with the my third "Highway Hypodermics" book, which has the subtitle of "On The Road Again." This edition has a lot of the things that were in the 2007 edition, with the added aspects of traveling as an LPN/ LVN, Allied Health traveling, and travel nursing when you are coming from other countries. All of the nursing stories are new and the travel company profiles have been updated, including several new companies!

Travel Nursing Goals

Living the dream... As I traveled the Oregon Coast last summer I was reminded about how fortunate I am to be living the dream of traveling across the United States and seeing some of the most awesome landscapes in the world. It leads me to wonder what dreams other traveling nurses have and how they are accomplishing their goals.

My first dream when I got into this profession was to travel along the Pacific Coast Highway in my Mustang convertible. Although I don't have the Mustang any longer, I did make it down the California coast with it before the engine gave out. When I was on assignment in Washington state, I finally completed my Highway 1/101 loop from the Seattle area around the Washington State peninsula all the way down to San Diego.

As I was discussing my travel plans with some of the other travel nurses that I work with, one of them mentioned that they have a goal of visiting all the national parks in the United States.

Other simple travel goals are to tour the coasts for lighthouses or covered bridges.

Other nurses have goals of seeing their grandchildren, being close to other family members, or finding a new place to live.

Are you just roaming around the United States, or do you have goals? If not, I challenge you to write you down some short term-goals and long-term goals.

My short-term goal was to travel the Pacific Coast highway. In the long run, I want to travel through all of the states. As of writing this, I still lack the states east of Wisconsin and the states North of Maryland.

The Baby Boomers

The age of the baby boomer is upon us and as these middle-aged Americans age, so does the demand for nurses to take care of them. The only problem with this demand is the supply, since not as many young men and women are entering the field of nursing as a career.

The median age for nurses in a 1990 study was about forty-five. Not that these nurses are invaluable in their more experienced years, but who is going to take their place when they decide to retire and travel fulltime without having to work?

In today's society the numbers of retiring nurses outnumber the nurses who are graduating from nursing school by 20%. I also know plenty of more experienced nurses who now use their knowledge to the best of their ability by consulting. Just because they are older and their legs don't work so well after forty years of running up and down hallways doesn't mean that their brain is lame also!

Working Conditions

After all, why would someone want to go into a profession where you are begged to work overtime so you can hear from the families a confirmation of the fact that nurses don't have time to take care of patients the way they should. Families are, however, somewhat more tolerant of it because they know that "all hospitals are short-staffed."

Why would you want to run around "like a chicken with its head cut off" for six hours before you get time to stop long enough to get a drink, go to the restroom, and grab a sandwich on your way back because we can't waste time for lunch? That abscess has to be drained!

Why would someone want to get into a profession where your feet are abused by all the long hours spent traipsing down the corridors of illness? If you are not one of the lucky ones to marry a foot masseur, you'd better learn self-message techniques and get some comfortable shoes.

Why would anyone want to spend time wiping butts, giving enemas, taking blood, then giving some back, cleaning up vomit, and my personal favorite—cleaning up that stringy sputum!

I am expected to work long hours, contend with ridiculous staffing circumstances, be treated like a dog by the administration, be yelled at by the physicians while dodging the clipboard, and be ridiculed by my nursing colleagues because I am definitely not working as hard as they are and I am not as good as they are.

I never could understand the old saying, "Nurses always eat their young," but that is what exactly we do. The new graduates are inexperienced and "stupid" because they haven't been around the block like we have, but I drag myself out of bed at 4:00 a.m. every morning because I care about the patients I take care of. I don't know why anybody wouldn't want to live the dream of being a nurse!

Career nurses are nurses because we are dedicated to our profession—because we really are concerned about patient care and the health of others. It is just hard to convey to someone else that this profession really does have its high points. If only they could see the patient's son who gives us a hug because we took care of his mother so well as she slipped from this life to the next. If only they could visit with the patient who went into ventricular fibrillation before my eyes and told me "thank you" ten minutes after I had defibrillated her. Making a difference in someone else's life—*that,* my friend is what nursing is all about.

Another concern for professional nurses is the issue of mandatory overtime. My colleague Melissa James stated, "After working a twelve-hour day shift at the nursing home, the night shift nurse called in. I was then informed by the director of nursing that I would stay or be turned into the state for patient abandonment."

Once being coerced into working those extra shifts, the nurses recognize in their hearts that they should not be touching syringes, handing out medications, or providing medical treatment, but they carry on as instructed because they have a family to feed at home and a nursing license to protect.

Investigative reports show that insomnia has some bearing on more than just a few aspects of nursing implementation, leading to sluggish responses, delayed reaction times, failure to make a start when appropriate, erroneous functions, decelerated thoughts, and a diminished recollection of nursing actions already performed.

Another factor influencing the nursing shortage is the increase of government interventions. With the rules and regulations of Medicare, medical treatment is ruled by money, not by patient need. This also is a factor with insurance entities, including HMOs, PPOs, and private insurance.

The patient's length of stay is governed by the patient's DRG (Diagnostic Related Group). If you have a hernia surgery, the government, not the physicians, tell you when your time is up. As a nurse, this bothers me terribly, because I see repeat patients that should have been taken care of longer the first time, who have been discharged only to return two weeks later with a severe infection and wound dehis-cence.

Who wants to work with people who have new diseases like vancomycin resistance enterococci (VRE), methicillin resistance staphylococcus aureus (MRSA), AIDS, HIV, tuberculosis, hepatitis, and other life-threatening contagious diseases?

Educational Factor

It does take money and time to get a nursing education. You find yourself having to work at least part-time and fitting study time in at 10:00 p.m. after everyone else is tucked in.

The year I went to nursing school I drove an hour and fifteen minutes to school, stayed all day at school, and then drove back home. Once home, I would change into my nursing assistant uniform just in time to help feed thirty patients and put them to bed. It was only after my job was finished that I went home and studied. Working only four hours a day meant a major cut in pay, but I worked the weekends also to bring home enough money to pay the bills and keep my insurance by working at least thirty-two hours in a week.

Even if you do find the money to attend nursing school, thousands of potential nursing students are turned down from nursing schools every year, not because they aren't smart or can't make the grade, but because there is no one to teach them. The fact of the matter is that a staff nurse with an associate's degree makes much more than a teaching nurse with a master's degree.

According to www.salary.com, a staff nurse in my hometown makes an average of $54,479, while an Instructor of Nursing makes

$42,408. That is a 33% decrease in salary after you go to school for four more years. What part of this makes sense? It doesn't, and that is why we can't get good instructors in our colleges to help provide more nurses for the working world.

Legal groups are in the process of advocating better salaries and benefits for nursing instructors. These groups are involved in the long process of working with state and federal government to pass laws that will give additional money to schools to increase the salaries of teachers. Health-related corporations have campaigns to encourage people to go into nursing and supply scholarships. Other schools are networking with more hospitals to make room to educate nurses; still, not enough is being done to help make a big difference in bringing nurses into the field.

Burn Out and Job Satisfaction

Burn-out in nursing is very common. Nurses get in a rut of working the same hospital for years and years and get to the point of being so stressed out that they start to blame others for things that go wrong, have a depressed affect, feel very irritable and frustrated all the time, and even have a short temper, a sense of powerlessness, and a very negative attitude about their work. They hate their work, and they literally have to "drag" themselves to work everyday.

What makes the situation even worse is that for the every one burned-out nurse there are three others that are around her. The burnout feeds itself into a raging fire that can destroy a unit and a nurse if it isn't carefully contained. Nurses are very dissatisfied in their jobs, and misery loves company. Soon staff morale is at an all-time low.

As a traveling nurse, things change with enough frequency that you don't get burned out, related to the fact that a fire can't get to raging stage if you are moving your fire every thirteen weeks. It doesn't have a chance to grow from a small campfire into a gigantic bonfire.

If you don't like the position you are in, travel nurses can just pick up camp and move on. Staff nurses have a tendency to stay in the same job for years and fight the burnout because they have settled into that geographical location because of family or friends. Most commonly, the way out is to leave the hospital or clinical situation and go into management, education, home health, or a physician's office. When they leave the floor, the nursing shortage then increases.

Conclusion

Let's face it, without a nursing shortage there would not be travel nursing. I'm all for better patient care and easing the nursing shortage, and that is why I take my turn helping out those hospitals in need. I don't get bored in the same old routine because I change hospitals, and even floors, every three to six months. No, travel nursing is not for everyone, but after reading this book you can make a more informed decision on whether or not travel nursing is right for you.

Chapter Two

What It Takes To Be a Travel Nurse

Some of the adjectives used to describe a traveling nurse are caring, adaptable, professional, accepting of criticism, positive attitude, ethical, and competent with the ability to live in a sometimes lonely world and in a small space. If you can fit into this mold, please read on to find out about the other qualities a travel nurse most possess.

Accepting Criticism

In travel nursing, you must be able to accept criticism. You are going into a jungle of many different animals, and if you are the meek little domestic tabby nurse, then you are going to be eaten alive. You are the one making the big bucks, and some will have the expectation that you have to be perfect. When you aren't perfect, someone *will* tell you about it.

When someone approaches you with something that makes them angry enough for them to tell you about it, you first need to ask them to talk to you when the time and place is appropriate. Invite them to sit down with you at lunch and discuss their problem with you.

After they voice their opinion about why they are upset with you, then ask for specific examples of what exactly you have done to cause the problem.

Actively listen to what they are saying. Are they putting you down to lift themselves up, or is it something that you could actually improve on? Are they rambling on just to hear themselves talk, or are they actually making sense? What is their motive?

Consider the source, also. There are people who will gripe about anything and everything, and then there are some people who would never complain about anything. Those gripers usually aren't hard to spot. Are they criticizing you only, or everyone else too?

After you have heard what they have to say, begin to separate fact from fiction and important from trivial. Is what they are saying going to matter in a week? Is what they are saying going to matter in a month? Will it make a change in your nursing career?

Keep all the useful information, and discard all the trivial and useless rambling. For instance, in the Emergency Department you may not be the fastest nurse, but you have to be the safest. Take the suggestions of others to improve your speed by improving on your time management skills. Learn how other nurses improve their time management to make your time management better.

Discard all the negative feelings. Have you ever worked with a charge nurse who all she ever did was charge? These people may seem to be bossy and griping all the time about not getting things done the way they think they should be done. No matter what they say, you have to discard the negative feelings. You are doing the best job that you can. As long as you know that you are doing your best, keep in the frame of mind that they are just attempting to guide you and help you remember what you need to do. If it seems that you are always the one getting yelled at and none of the other staff, then you need to bring that up to your recruiter or nurse manager.

Have a sense of humor with these types of people when appropriate. When people ask me, "Where have you been?" My favorite come back is "Down the hall eating Bon-Bons and drinking diet soda." Duh! Where do they really think I have been? I'm down the hallway with my patients. Then I inform them of what I have been doing and what I'm fixing to do.

Help others learn to give praise along with criticism. There have been times when I have asked, "And exactly what have I done right today?"

Push them into giving you a positive comment. If they can't give you a positive comment, then you can classify that criticism session a "gripe session" and that person is purely just complaining to have something to do.

As a traveler, you will go into units with definite problems. If they didn't have any big problems, they would have staff that wanted to be there and they wouldn't need you. You must be motivated by the criticism and not let them manipulate you with their analysis. Take what you can to improve yourself and let the other stuff roll off of your back.

The biggest difference in accepting criticism as a staff nurse and as a traveler is that you feel like you are out there all by yourself. It's you against the world. If you aren't strong enough to take it, you will be miserable.

Getting Along With Others

Remember in grade school when we had this spot on our report cards that read, "Gets along and plays well with others?" Well, that is about how things are in the big world also.

Your first impression takes you a long ways when it comes to getting along and working well with others upon arrival to your new unit. Go to your charge nurse the first day with a smile and tell them who you are and that, "I'm here to help." Remember that it is awfully hard to chew on someone's butt when they are smiling.

A slightly aggressive approach here is much better than one in which you saunter up to the nurses' station and just sit there. That may give the first impression that you are lazy and just want to sit around instead of being excited to help, and being excited about your new adventure.

Be optimistic that this assignment is going to be the best you have ever had. This is your home floor for the next few months, so don't go onto the floor with an attitude of "What kind of mess did I get myself into?" The unit may be an older unit, but even older units can have great staffs.

Whatever you do, don't be late on your first day. When you first get into town, drive the route several times to get an idea of how long it is going to take to get from your apartment to the hospital. Then add ten minutes to make sure that you get there early.

In the first week of orientation, it is very important to remember that you have two ears and only one mouth. Don't say all the things that you can do, but show them what you can do. Take an active roll in orientation and promote your own independence. One of the easiest ways to do this is to answer call lights without being told to, and do it very promptly. This will show others that you have a willingness to work.

Take the focus off of yourself when people start asking about your background by also being interested in what they have to say. Sometimes the background of others can be just as exciting as traveling around the United States taking care of people. I have run into fascinating nurses who have lived in some of the places that I have worked at, nurses who lived in the same type of farm that my grandparents lived on, and nurses who are new not only to nursing, but to the United States.

After working there for a few weeks, both you and the other nurses get more relaxed and comfortable with each other, but you still have to remember about having two ears and one mouth. This is the easiest time to mess things up by bragging about all the things you have done. Just remember that life is not a box of chocolates, but a jar of jalapeño's that can burn your butts later.

When conflict comes up, you have to use it as a tool for input instead of a tool of destruction. Don't feed into the negative thoughts of others and join into the conflicts that already exist on the floor. Although you might have a few suggestions, it isn't wise to express them until you have settled in and can confide in a charge nurse or unit manager who really wants to know what you think.

Avoid negative feelings about others and remember that we are all different. Each one of us can bring something to the table to make a positive impact on the unit; you just have to use a lot more tact than you would if you were a regular floor nurse.

Keep opinions that will cause an emotional outburst to yourself. A highly emotional situation can bring up some very bad tempers. When emotions, instead of facts, come out in a conflict, you have gone too far.

As a staff nurse, you might get along with some nurses but still have a few sparse friends or a cliché that sees things the way you do, but remember, as a traveling nurse you will soon be alienated if you are too far out of the mold. An alienated nurse will never have a fun assignment.

Professionalism

A traveler must be professional. As soon as you walk into the hospital and onto your unit, your professionalism is what people see. Do you walk with your head up or down? Professionalism is probably the most critical factor in making or breaking a travel assignment.

You have to remember that no one knows you when you arrive. You have to prove to those around you that you are not going from assignment to assignment because you can't get any other nursing job. You have to prove that you are a traveling nurse because you want to be a traveling nurse.

The first step to professionalism is the way you look. It's not mandatory, but having your hair up off your shoulders is a good start. Have it neatly trimmed and pulled back nicely. Make sure that your uniform is nice and clean without wrinkles. I know that should be a given, but you would be surprised at how many times I have seen unkempt uniforms.

During orientation, be alert to their policies and procedures. If you have questions, don't be afraid to ask. Do not just go off and do things your own way. Ask your preceptor questions about how they accomplish certain tasks. Never say, "Well, I can't do it that way because it isn't what I learned in nursing school." Get out the policy and procedure book to find out how the facility management wants it done. You also don't want to say, "You need to do it this way, because this is the way we did it in Florida."

Although there are times when the nurses take it upon themselves to take a short cut, it is then that you will need to use your nursing judgment. For example, don't break sterile field just because the OR tech is doing it. Don't suction a tracheostomy without using sterile technique just because the respiratory therapist says it really not necessary.

By asking the preceptor or charge nurse how they do things, you will be perceived as one who cares about doing things the right way. The staff will have confidence in your skills.

As a traveler, it is really tough to "tell" people of certain top-notch skills that you may have, like starting those hard to get IVs. No matter how much you tell them, the only way people will ultimately believe in your skills is by proving your skills to them.

Another aspect of professionalism is that you must not get involved in the unit's politics. After all, isn't that one of the reasons we travel? The easiest way of doing this is by not hanging out at the nurses' station, talking about tummy tucks, boob jobs, and boyfriends. You need to be down the hallway with your patients. Patient care has to be number one.

In my first year of traveling, I was in a situation where there were two of us travelers taking care of the same patient. I was really having a tough time keeping up with a patient that demanded a lot of my attention; therefore, I took my charts down to the far end of the hallway closer so I could do more frequent checks. I survived the night with the patient in good shape and gave my report to the other traveler.

When I came back to work, I found that the other traveler stayed up at the nurses' station, chatting with everyone for an hour, and the patient got into trouble. They ended up terminating her contract over the deal, but not before she blamed the whole thing on me. Luckily, I had obtained a second opinion on the person from my charge nurse, who went to bat for me, telling the unit manager that I had spent all night not far from the patient. If I had spent all night up at the nurses' station talking with the others or spent my time in another unprofessional way, the outcome may have been much different for me.

Competency

Along with professionalism comes competency. The first thing you might think of is taking tests to prove your competence. Yes, we have already done that to become nurses, but as a traveling nurse you will have to prove yourself over and over again.

On just about every nursing assignment that I have been on in the past two years I have had to take a medication test. If you will just take time to look over the drug book and know all of the most common medications, like coumadin, lasix, lovenox, and your narcotics, along with knowing your conversion factors, drip rates, and metric system, you should be okay. Yeah, I know... sometimes easier said that done. Also, you have to know the common antidotes, such as Vitamin K, Protamine, and Narcan.

They have also come up with a clinical-based test called the "Performance Based Development System." In this test you are rated on situational performance.

This test has been used for quite some time, and although some believe that is totally unfair, it is something that traveling nurses are going to have to face at some point, unless you boycott all the hospitals that do this type of testing. Just be prepared and knowledgeable of its existence. It will be explained in more detail in a later chapter.

Adaptability And Flexibility

This is a biggie for travel nurses. If you cannot accept change easily, don't even think about being a travel nurse. "Yes, but I need the money." No amount of money is going to be worth the amount of misery you will put yourself through.

The first adaptation you will encounter is a new place to live. Housing can be very different, depending on your location. You can't have a penthouse suite in the Trump Tower that is as big as a barn. Most living arrangements are small apartments, from 600-900 square feet, with a minimal amount of furniture.

Or it could be an extended-stay hotel or corporate housing. It might even be just a single hotel room. Can you live in such a small space for three months? As long as it is clean, I could do anything for a few months, but after that I would be looking for a new place to go. Some companies will let you find alternative housing, but for others there may be no alternative. In some seasonal areas you will find this a big problem: California in vegetable harvest or Florida, Arizona, or Southern California during the winter.

The next adaptability issue is orientation to the hospital and units. Orientation is done several ways. I have done five days general and hospital orientation before getting to the floor to one-day general and one-day nursing orientation, to four hours of floor orientation to orientation online. However long orientation is, use it to your advantage. This is usually thought of as a hospital's way to get you to think that they are the best, but it can also be a great time to meet other travelers.

Learn as much as you can about the resources available to you. How do you solve problems? What community resources are available to your patients? What educational resources are available to you? Get yourself a three-ring binder and put all of your facility information in it to carry with you. It is also a good idea to get a phone list of the numbers you will use frequently, such as the lab, pharmacy, radiology, and the staffing office. As a traveler, once you have memorized this list it's time to move on.

Once you get to the floor, your orientation can be anywhere from one hour to three days. This is the reason why one of the qualifications for being a travel nurse is one year of experience. As a traveler, you are expected to hit the floor running.

The most common scenario is to follow someone that first day to learn the routine of the floor and the second day take a few patients yourself. The third day you need to be on your own, with someone as a resource person. After your first orientation week you will be on your own, and it's then that you have to fly by yourself, but do not be afraid to ask questions about hospital policy and procedure.

Orientation is also an excellent time to ask the education department what will be available to you during the next three months. Take time out to learn more about educational opportunities. You will be surprised at how much education is available to travelers for free or a small fee.

Once you get on the unit you are going to have to adapt to their way of doing things. As a traveler, the phrase you need to repeat the most is "How do you do things here?" The simple fact is that if you follow the policy and procedures of that unit and that particular hospital, you will be much better off than if you go and do things on your own. It is when you start to act like it's going to be your way or the highway that things can turn around from being pleasant to everyone being hostile towards you. You have to blend in without compromising nursing ethics.

Another aspect of adaptability is the issue of "floating." As a traveler, you will be expected to float, and in some hospitals, you will be the first one to float. It is just part of the job.

What isn't part of the job is floating to a unit in which you have had no orientation to, or no experience in. That is why you need to protect yourself by putting into your contract what floors you can float to. Other than that, you need to float to your areas of competency with a smile and a positive attitude. Say to yourself, "I'm just here to help," because that is really what a traveler is—a person who has been hired by the facility to help out in a time of need.

If you don't feel that you are competent to float to a certain area, discuss it with the house supervisor. Although you know your areas of competency and it's in your contract, most likely the one making the decision doesn't know that. Tell them the areas you are comfortable with and the areas with which you are not comfortable. I have found that this may entail describing not only the type of floor, but the type of patient as well. I don't mind going to the Intensive Care Unit for low level patients, but I cannot and will not take a patient with an arterial line or ventilator because I haven't been trained to maintain patients with that type of equipment, but I can take a post heart catheter patient or one that just requires extra attention because of a drip that they are receiving.

The thing that helps me out the most with floating is remembering the basics: assessment, plan, implementation, evaluation and documentation. It doesn't matter if I am on the rehab unit, medical unit, psychiatric unit, or emergency department; the basics of assessment and planning are always the same; it is the area of implementation that causes some difficulty.

Ask the charge nurse the minute you get to the floor the basics of the patients that you are expected to take care of. If you have any concerns at all about the type of patient, or if you are uncomfortable in taking care of that patient, you need to express that to the charge nurse, and do *not* accept report for that patient. You cannot abandon a patient if you never took responsibility for that patient by taking report.

It can get tough out there, but remember that patient safety must come first. When it gets tough, you have to stick up for yourself and remember that the house supervisor or charge nurse is not going to be standing there with you in front of the state nursing board if things go wrong.

The Lonely Road

You have to adjust to loneliness on the road. My husband and our son travel with me, but there are times when I still feel some loneliness on the road—loneliness for my parents, my brother, and friends that I have left behind.

Loneliness can be combated by creating more adventure. Get to know the other travelers, and plan outings together. Even exploring by yourself can be great fun. I often get into my truck and head down the highway, seeing all the sites in solitude.

The first weekend go south, the next go north, go west and east on subsequent weekends and just drive to see what is out there. For example, the first weekend that I was here in Southern Florida I drove to the beach in Hollywood and then drove south to Miami Beach. The next weekend I went back to Hollywood Beach and then drove the coastal highway north to Palm Beach. When my parents came down to visit, we headed west and went to the Everglades. My next trips, hopefully, will be to north Orlando and Cape Canaveral.

As for family, I keep in touch via my cell phone and email. If you don't have a cell phone, this is a good time to get one. In fact, I didn't have one until I went on the road. With the free minutes in the evening, I could call home every day if I so desired.

Another great way to keep in touch with family is through the Internet. It is also a great place to meet other traveling nurses with chat and discussion forums such as Delphi Traveling Nurses and Therapy and Ultimate Nurse Forums. I had a blast at the Delphi meet-and-greet that I attended in New Orleans. I post a lot of pictures online also, so my family feels like they have a connection with me.

Another way to combat loneliness is to join a local club or organization such as a sports club, fitness center, church organization, friends of the library, etc. There are plenty of places to reach out for friends, but you will still have those times when you are all by yourself, and you will feel the pit of loneliness.

In the times when there is no one to reach out to, I would suggest spending those moments writing in a journal. Write about your nursing career, write about how you are feeling, or write about where you want to go in your future.

In Conclusion

Travel nursing can be a very rewarding career if you truly have what it takes. If you are professional, credible, can stand up for yourself, adapt to many situations, float to different floors, live in a small space without many friends, and do all of this with a positive attitude, then I invite you to read on and enjoy the prospects of a great new career as a traveling nurse.

Chapter Three

The Good, the Bad, and the Ugly

"Along the fairways of life, you must stop and smell the roses; for you only get to play one round."

That is one of my favorite golf quotes from one of the greatest players ever: Ben Hogan. In travel nursing, sometimes you play a long par five in a twenty-six-week contract, while others are shorter par four thirteen weekers or par three eight week contracts. Either way, the journey is full of roses, along with a few thorns. And yes, at times we run completely off course and into the lake, but swing back to the shore and travel on down the road.

What does all this have to do with travel nursing? The road traveled has many rewards, but it also has its drawbacks, and it even can throw us completely off-course with an ugly disaster.

Making New Friends

Don't look at your travel assignment as being a lonely adventure; rather look at it as an opportunity to make new friends in new places. Orientation is the first place to make new friends. Find out who the other travelers are. During orientation, try to find out more information about them, like where they are from, where they have been, and what type of hobbies they have. Make an attempt to take your lunch breaks together.

During the nursing orientation, it is interesting how the travelers usually find each other and do things together from the start. The travelers are the ones who have seen the equipment at other hospitals and can give help if a new staff member has not seen the equipment.

Try to get the other travelers' email addresses, and after a while, trade phone numbers. You can give some hint about the area of town you live in, but don't push the exact address or they might think that you are out to stalk them, and vise versa, in that you don't know what type of person they really are. Just by giving out simple information you can deduct if the person lives in your complex. In several situations I have found that if there are only a few apartment complexes that accept short-term leases, you will probably find other travel nurses in the same complex as you are in.

Other places to meet people are at social functions, such as church groups or friends of the library. Usually there is also some kind of pet or zoo group if the outdoors is your thing. Take your dog to the dog park and meet others there.

If you are on the Internet, there are plenty of travel nursing groups. I frequent the Delphi Forums Travel Nursing groups, and have been to several meet-and-greets. These meetings are great fun and easily found in the higher traveled areas such as Southern Florida, Phoenix, San Francisco, and some New England regions.

Selecting Assignments Where You Desire

No one else can tell you where to go as a travel nurse—well, not unless you're married. You are free to fly with the wind to the most exotic and out-of-the-way places like the rural areas of Oklahoma, Texas, Nebraska or Iowa, or enjoy an assignment in the metropolis of New York City, Miami, Los Angeles, or Phoenix. Travel to the beaches of Southern California, Atlantic City or Hawaii. Assignments can also be found ranging in areas from the Virgin Islands to the great state of Alaska.

You might have to change companies, but so far I have gone every place that I have wanted to visit. This is easier done if you have more than one specialty, like medical intensive care, surgical intensive care, cardiovascular intensive care, and emergency room, or telemetry, medical, surgical, step-down and rehab.

What other career will allow you to be a snowbird when you are thirty-five years old instead of sixty-five years old? When it comes time to make a move, my husband selects what state he would like to go to, then I put my state into the mixture and we submit to those hospitals and see who gives us the best deal. My son would have a choice, but he just wants to go to Washington, where his girlfriend is. For the summer, I wanted Nebraska and hubby wanted Iowa; we went to Iowa. For the winter, I wanted Florida, hubby wanted southern Texas: I'm writing this chapter in Florida. And yes, next summer we plan on spending it in Washington State.

Miniature Vacations

One of my favorite aspects of travel nursing is the mini-vacations. These are little two nights away to some place a little farther than you could go on a day trip.

When I was in Central California, my family and I went to San Francisco one day then up the Pacific coast highway to the Redwoods. The first night we stayed at a small motel on the outskirts of San Francisco in an older fishing village.

The second night we stayed in the Redwoods. The trees were gorgeous, with their red and green colors. The Redwood Trail is also the site of the road picture on my first travel nursing book, *Highway Hypodermics: Your Road Map to Travel Nursing*.

While on assignment in Iowa, we toured the bridges of Madison County and John Wayne's birthplace on one road trip, and later made a trip to Minneapolis, Minnesota to watch the Twins play baseball and visit the Mall of America.

One assignment in Tupelo, Mississippi not only took us to the site of Elvis's birthplace, but a day adventure took us to the place where he lived and died, at Graceland, in Memphis, Tennessee. On a bigger adventure, we spent some time a week before Christmas at the Opryland Hotel in Nashville and had the extraordinary experience of Christmas in Nashville. While in Nashville we explored many sites, such as the Ryman Auditorium, the Country Music Hall of Fame, and took in a show at the Grand Ole Opry.

See The United States

When I started out as a traveling nurse, I had been east of the Mississippi River once, and that was for less than twenty-four hours. Now I can say that I have not only crossed the mighty Mississip, but I have even made it to the Eastern Time Zone. In the last two years alone I have been from the beaches of Pismo, California to Southern Miami Beach, and from the swamps of Louisiana to the lakes of Minnesota.

If water and beaches are not your thing, then how about an amazing sunset in the Arizona sky? Or you can take in the breathtaking view from the top of the Colorado mountains.

How about a goal of seeing all the National Parks that the United States has to offer? You can visit the Everglades, the Appalachians, The Rocky Mountains, Yellowstone, The Grand Canyon, and Yosemite.

Are you into history? How about a trip through the history of the United States, from Washington D.C. to the Battle of New Orleans, the Battle of Shiloh, or the Alamo. Don't forget to visit the many military museums, including the Smithsonian, the Air Force Museum in Pensacola, FL, and there are several battleships to visit.

Control Of Your Destination

Only you can choose your final destination. Although some recruiters attempt to get you to go where they want you to go, you are the one who has the final say. Well, unless your travel with a family, like I said before, and then it can be a fun adventure for all. Take a family vote and discuss it together as to where everyone would like to go.

Keep your eyes and ears out for interesting places to visit by networking with other travel nurses. Others might have ideas of great places they have been to that you may have never thought of.

Depending on your specialty, you may be somewhat limited, but you will always have a choice, even if it means changing companies. If you have a low-demand specialty like NICU, Pediatrics, Psychiatric, or Rehab, then it is a good idea to keep your file up-to-date with three to five different companies.

Whether it is a small town, bustling city, or moderate city in the Midwest, you will always have the final say on where you will spend the next thirteen weeks.

Explore Before You Make The Big Move

Taking a travel assignment in a place where you think you would like to permanently move to is an excellent idea. It is much easier to decide if you would like to make a big move after you have had a trial period of eight to thirteen weeks.

You can spend the entire time on your assignment exploring the community, from parks, recreation, city leaders, major employers, crime rate, and the best parts of the city. This time can also be spent looking for a house to live in permanently.

What about the best nursing jobs? You will have several options to explore, including permanent staffing, per diem work, or an available float pool.

If you have children, this will give you time to explore educational options. Is there a magnet school that your child would fit into? What is the best junior high or high school? Contact any local educational organizations such as the Parent-Teacher Association. You can also visit schools after narrowing your choices down to a few good ones.

If the city or town isn't exactly what you thought it would be, it is much easier to pick up and move when your assignment is done than if you had moved your entire household to the new area.

Unlimited Field Trips

If you live in the same place for years, how often do you visit the zoo or the local museum? You think that they have the same old exhibits, and it is true that some of the exhibits do not change, but as a traveling nurse the exhibits at a museum or zoo are always changing. New things are abundant. As a travel nurse, you will not only have an opportunity to see a lot of new arrivals at the zoo, but opportunities to take a multitude of other field trips to see new things.

You do not even need a child to go to the zoo to learn about nature. You can find plenty of opportunities outside the hustle and bustle of the big city for all kinds of nature activities.

Don't feel like taking a hike? Go to the lake or park and just watch the birds and look for fish in the shallow water. This is an excellent time to take up the hobby of photography.

Civil War and other natural history sites are also great for a field trip. A lot of the nature sites have recorded information at a touch of a button. On the battlefield, you push the button and hear the sound of war. You can "see" the big cannons going off and feel the earth shake as men fight for freedom.

Nursing Freedom

Travel nursing affords you the luxury of being in total control of your nursing career and decisions. You can be a rural nurse, a big city nurse, or even have endless educational opportunities at a teaching hospital.

You can be a level-one trauma nurse, or you can experience the adventure of a rural emergency room. In fact, some of the most interesting cases I have seen were at a small hospital in the emergency room. The excitement happens more often in a trauma center, but you would be amazed at what can happen out in the middle of nowhere.

As an intensive care nurse, with the proper training you can go from a small ICU that does ventilators and drips, to a large university hospital where everyone has an arterial line and a balloon pump.

You have total control of your destination, from water skiing in the summer to snow skiing in the winter, or not ever having to see snow again. Take life easy in rural Iowa or pump up the jams on Miami Beach.

You can choose the length of your contract. Although most contracts are thirteen weeks, several eight-week and twenty-six week contracts can be found. You can also choose the number of renewals that you accept.

Endless Educational Opportunities

Just because you are traveling doesn't mean that the learning has to stop. In fact, the educational opportunities increase, related to the fact that with every change in assignment you get a new list of classes available.

Usually, orientation is organized by the educational department. This is a prime opportunity to get a list of classes that will be offered during the next three months of your contract. Sometimes you might have to pay a fee, but that is a very small price to pay for higher education. There are a lot of places that will let you take the classes for free.

Always be on the lookout for continuing education programs at other nearby hospitals or universities. Some agencies even have a deal worked out with places online for you to get your educational opportunities through online courses.

You can also get an advanced degree online while on assignment. There are plenty of programs available through universities, and the list grows by leaps and bounds each year.

The ultimate educational assignment would be at a teaching hospital. All kinds of classes are available at these hospitals, and you might even like the area so well that you stay and get an advanced degree.

Enhance Your Resumé

A lot of nurses are concerned that being a traveling nurse will make their resum-é look like they can't hold a good job, when in actuality it can have just the opposite effect in that it can show that you are well diversified and adaptable.

Stability can be shown in many different ways, including staying with the same company and renewing contracts. No, neither of these are a "have to." I know plenty of travelers who have to change companies because they are in a specialty in which jobs are few and far between; therefore changing companies at times is a necessity to find jobs.

Travel nursing assignments can also show your ability to adapt to new situations with little orientation. It shows that you can stand on your own two feet in the midst of a brand new situation.

Most importantly, it shows that you are not afraid of change, and that you welcome change with open arms.

Better Pay

A lot of nurses travel due to the better pay. Staff nurses around the country are averaging between twenty and thirty-five dollars per hour, but traveling nurses make an average of twenty-five to forty-five dollars per hour, depending on the location and specialty. Generally speaking, the travel nurse gets 20% more than the staff nurse. Along with this increase in pay, travel expenses are also paid for. This will give extra money to get caught up on other bills, such as credit cards.

Not only does your pay increase, but all income related to travel and per diem are non-taxable by using the tax advantage. This means that in the right circumstances, up to half of your pay could be non-taxable. This means that you save big bucks when it comes to your taxes. It is not uncommon for a traveling nurse to save three to five thousand dollars on taxes. This, of course, all hinges on the fact that you have a "tax home" (which we will discuss in a later chapter).

Regional Food

Now that we have made more money, we want to eat new things! The United States has a wide variety of foods, whether you're in the Southeast, Southwest, Northeast, Northwest, Midwest, or Central Plains.

San Francisco is a must-stop for sourdough bread. In fact, give me some clam chowder in a sourdough bowl while I'm sitting on the pier watching the seals lounge around anytime.

The East is famous for the shrimp burgers that can be found in North Carolina, Brunswick Stew, Boston Baked Beans, and a "dog" from Coney Island.

Florida is best known not only for it's key lime pie, but other tropical and swamp favorites such as mango chicken and fried alligator.

In the south you will find a great combination of fried chicken, mashed potatoes, gravy, and cornbread, along with some fiery Cajun jambalaya, etouffee, and blackened catfish.

The Midwest is known for its home-grown corn and beef. Some of the best barbeque can be found in the Kansas and Missouri regions, along with the best steaks coming out of Nebraska.

A trip to the Southwest will bring you the best in Tex-Mex, chilis, burritos, and other flavors with a kick, which are influenced by our neighbors to the south.

Choice In Housing

Now that your tummy is full, you will need a place to rest your head. The choices are many when it comes to housing.

The least expensive that I have found is to travel in a recreational vehicle. There is plenty of money left over after your housing stipend. Some people purchase larger recreational vehicles (RVs) and use the housing stipend to pay for the RV, while others purchase an RV outright, with no RV payment, and pocket the extra money from the housing stipend. There is no room service at an RV park and the space is small, but you can enjoy the great outdoors.

The most popular housing option is an apartment. Your travel agency will find a one-bedroom apartment for you to stay in, or if you travel with your family, a two-bedroom can usually be found. Some companies will charge you extra for the added space, but companies are becoming more and more flexible with housing needs. Although we are seeing a trend in some of the more desirable places in which housing is decreasing, du to the fact that apartment complexes are being turned into condominiums. Furniture packages are standard with most companies, but do not hesitate to ask about a customized furniture package or other options.

Another option that has to be used sometimes is hotels or extended stays. Those are somewhat more expensive, but you do have the luxury of a housekeeper. Pots, pans, linens, microwaves, and televisions are usually included in these types of housing units.

Responsibility

The great thing about traveling is that I am responsible for only my actions and choices in my career.

There is no corporate ladder to climb. I do not have to bust my hinny to prove my worthiness as a managerial candidate.

Most of the time someone else is in charge; therefore, I don't have to worry about what the other nurses are doing either. I just have to keep track of what I am doing.

I go to work and find more emphasis on the responsibility of taking care of my patients. I am responsible for myself and my actions towards my patients.

Yes, I have to get along with others, but if someone gets angry towards me I don't have to work in a hostile environment for years and years...only three months. I am responsible for myself and soon I will leave them and their noxious attitude. I'm not responsible for the way others think.

If for some reason you make a physician mad at you in the middle of the night, after three months it won't matter because you'll be gone. You just have to worry about the patients.

Politics

If you are not into travel nursing as it relates to higher pay rates, then you are probably in it because you are sick and tired of all the politics you catch as a regular staff member.

As a traveler, you do not have to worry about who is going to get the unit manager position, who is going to be the next house supervisor, or who is going to get the holidays off. If I want the holidays off, then I just make sure that my contract ends on December 15th and schedule my next assignment to begin on January 15th.

You do not get attached to the other nurses enough to really get into the juicy gossip. Be kind and somewhat sociable, but don't get sucked into talking about other nurses, knocking the weird patient who is in the emergency room again or the married surgeon who is having an affair with the circulating nurse.

You have control of your contract. You can specify your patient-to-nurse ratio, what areas you will float to and what days you need off instead of having to go through a strike for better benefits, wages, and working conditions. You choose the company that is right for you, and if you find out that the company is no longer working for you, then you can change companies.

Going Away

Once you have spent a wonderful thirteen weeks at an assignment, there is usually some kind of going away celebration. Whether it's cake and ice cream or pizza delivery, usually something is planned; sometimes it is just a card and hugs. Even at my least favorite place we took pictures and had a few laughs.

In almost all assignments there has been someone with whom I have stayed in touch. I send Christmas cards to Arizona, California, Iowa, Oklahoma, and Mississippi.

My best going away was in California, where we had cake and ice cream, and then the nursing assistants and my licensed practical nurse gave me a rose. Potlucks are also very good; just don't be afraid to ask for the recipe of your favorite dish.

At times it is very hard to leave, but think of all the friends you have met along the way, and all the friendships that are yet to come.

Obtaining States' Licenses

It was the best of times, it was the worst of times, and it was the loneliness of times, with staff grudges, instability, licensing issues, and taxes. Yes, along with all the good that we have discussed so far come some of the bad times of traveling.

One nuisance is the time that it takes to get a new license in each state, and then having to decide whether or not to renew that license. What used to take a few hours to fill out and send in now sometimes can take days if you have to work with a police station that only does fingerprints on a certain day, and time consuming if the local place to get photos in thirty miles away. Not tough to do—just time consuming. And then, instead of renewing one license every two to four years, you may have several that need to be renewed, or you may need a new license for the next assignment.

This has become somewhat easier with the creation of the compact licensure system, but not even half of the states are "compact." This is a national coalition of states that recognize each other's licenses. The nurse has to be a resident of a compact state, then she can travel to other compact states without having to get a new license. For instance, since my home is in Idaho, my Idaho nursing license is a compact nursing license. When I went to Iowa, Arizona, and Mississippi, there was no need to get a new license; I just gave the hospital a copy of my Idaho license.

I also carry a few other states: California, where I worked for four years, Oklahoma, where my parents live, and Florida, a great spot for the winter. When it comes to renewal time, I will have four licenses that need to be renewed (CA, OK, ID, & FL). Unlike that, if I did not live in a compact state I would have Arizona, Iowa, Mississippi, and the four others, for a total of seven licenses that would come up for renewal. In any case, you need to decide which licenses you might use again, then put the others on an inactive status.

More information can be found about the different states and compact licensing in an upcoming chapter. Make sure that you call to see about the time factor when obtaining a new license.

Little or No Orientation

For travel nurses, a change is as good as a vacation, but change can also be traumatic to some nurses, especially the "newbies." Nurses start travel nursing because of the excitement and adventure, then they have to face the reality of catching on quickly and hitting the floor running.

The ideal traveler needs to be able to follow someone one day and take off on their own the next. At times, nursing orientation is as short as a few hours, while other orientations last for a week.

For instance, in Oklahoma City I had four hours of computer class and four hours of on-the-floor orientation, then I was on my own. In Plantation, Florida, I had five 8-hour days of orientation, then three days on the floor.

In some cases I have had the nursing managers ask me what type of orientation I am used to and go with my style of orientation, but others have their own way of doing things, and that is fine also. Part of being a travel nurse is being a fast learner and going with the flow. Personally, I want one day to follow and then let me go, but I know that others would like to have the full three days with someone else.

If you do not feel comfortable after your orientation, you need to talk to your manager about what you don't feel comfortable with, and then learn what you can look for next time to make your orientation go smoother and quicker. Just remember the basics of nursing: assessment, planning, implementation, evaluation, and follow-up.

Loneliness

It doesn't matter whether you travel alone or with a family, loneliness will find you.

I was recently in Fort Myers, Florida, meeting with two single travelers, and I posed the question to them, "How do you combat loneliness as a single traveler?" They both said to combat the loneliness they go shopping, including window shopping, spending time with pets, or just spend time outside at a park or beach and watch people.

I miss my family in Oklahoma, but have very strong ties in that I call my parents two to three times a week, and my brother every Tuesday. My husband calls his 90-year-old mother almost every day.

Take time to get involved in other activities such as a church, friends of the library, and network with other travelers. Keeping in touch is easy with a cell phone and/or a computer.

Instability

Assignments usually are thirteen weeks, with the option of renewing. By renewing a contract you can create some sense of stability.

When it comes to credit, a travel nurse can look volatile, but that can be combated by putting on your credit application that you have been a registered nurse for twelve years, or however long. Also, by staying with the same travel company you can create some stability for credit.

The extended time on the contract decreases the times you have to move each year and the number of orientations you have to attend. On the average, I move two to three times a year: once in the spring, once in the fall, with the possibility of one other if

I'm not too happy with either hospital that I have chosen that year.

States' Taxes

The next big worry about the different states you visit is with their state taxes. Along with the difference licensures in each state, each also has a different rate of state tax, from no state tax to almost 10% state tax. The states without an income tax include: Alaska, Florida, Nevada, South Dakota, Texas, Washington and Wyoming. Consequently, if you are a traveling nurse without any strong ties to a certain place, the best states to settle in related to tax rates and compact licensing are South Dakota and Texas.

Then you have California and Maryland, which not only have some of the highest tax rates, but if you are there for more than six to nine months you are considered a resident of the state, and you end up paying the high tax rate instead of a lower tax rate at your "tax home."

You may have to file in four different states, plus your state of residence, if you take only thirteen-week assignments and each of the assignments is in a different sate. You should get at least most of your non-residence state money back, but you will have to pay someone or buy a program for each state to file, or do things "the long way," with the paper forms. As a traveling nurse, I would not ever dream of doing things "the old fashioned" way of pen and calculator. Although a little higher priced than do-it- yourself type programs, tax advisors and preparers are worth their weight in gold if they specialize in traveling occupational taxes. We will discuss taxes more in a later chapter.

Once you know the state to which you are going to traveling, check out their website for tax information and any special rules.

Sick Days

Another downside related to money is losing out when you are not feeling so great. Not only do you not get paid for the day that you miss, but some companies even charge you for housing costs, their reason being that they are paying for housing for you to work thirty-six hours a week, and when you don't live up to that obligation, they do not get their money from their hospital bill rate; therefore, they are losing out on income, hence you will loose also.

Some of the smaller companies are starting to let nurses have paid time off and/or vacation pay, but this is a very new concept. Most companies that I have dealt with will require you to make those days up, either during that week or the next week. If a whole week is missed, the days may be added to the end of the contract.

If you are prone to sickness or have a long-term condition that flairs up from time to time, definitely get long-term, or at least short-term disability insurance.

Staff Grudges

Some of the ugliest situations I have seen are staff grudges. Now that you are making all these "big bucks," some regular staff think that you need to be assigned the most difficult patients, because travelers are there just for the money anyway.

There is also this misconception in some places that the hospital's bill rate (what they are paying out) is also what the nurses are getting; therefore, I have had some nurses want to know if I really do make fifty dollars an hour. They do not understand about the company getting their share and the travel company paying out for housing.

Some nurses have expressed the fact that they get the tough bed assignments because the staff believes that since the traveler makes more money, they can have the group of patients with persistent nausea, vomiting, diarrhea, the gastro-intestinal bleeds, and the Alzheimer's patients.

Traveler "hostile" hospitals are out there, but they are few and far between. I have only been in one hospital where the hospital management wasn't hostile, but the nurses were; and then again, the nurse management was also "relieved of duties" half way through the assignment.

Packing and Moving Every Three Months

This can be a very ugly problem if you can not pack lightly. My poor husband...I have to pick on him here. He is a pack rat, and this travel thing has been so stressful on him because he can't find all these "basement bargains" at the thrift store and bring them home. Of course I don't have a problem, since all I bring is all the office stuff and books. Now you know why I travel with a small cargo trailer.

Find out in advance what the apartment is going to come with. Sometimes you will have full linen and kitchen utensils if you are in corporate housing, but if you have an apartment, then these things usually aren't available. That is where the thrift store shopping comes in handy.

Most of the time, though, you will have a dresser, side table, and bed in the bedroom, with a couch and chair in the living room, with a dining room table and chairs in either the dining area or the kitchen. Don't forget to take your vacuum, a television, a microwave, and pot-holders.

What you pack and whom you travel with can also make a difference. For the three of us (me, my husband, and my son), we tend to travel a little heavy. We not only have the office stuff, but hubby has his "workshop" in the front of the trailer to do small repairs, along with all the son's books and schoolwork supplies. Not to mention the fact that we probably have way too many kitchen and cooking items.

Nowadays, I throw things out at the end of the assignment just so hubby can fulfill his thrift store treasure-shopping habit every three to six months. If there is a deal on housewares to be found, my husband can find it. The thrift stores are definitely a travel nurse's friend for supplies you need at the beginning of an assignment, then you get tax credits for turning things in at the end.

A lot of the travelers I have recently met either drive pickups with lockable shells or sport utility vehicles. It can be done in a car by choosing what you take carefully. Take a first assignment within a few hundred miles to get a good idea of what you need if you require a test run.

Moving companies are usually too expensive to help you move every time if you have a family, but it can be feasible to hire someone from a temporary agency to help unload your own trailer or a rental trailer, if need be.

In conclusion

There are many good things, a small amount of bad things, and few ugly things you should know about travel nursing. Your mission, should you choose to accept it, is to make a list of all the good and bad things that you need to consider to further evaluate if this way of life is right for you.

Travel nursing is definitely an adventure. You just have to be tough enough to take a few bumps in the road.

Chapter Four

Traveling As an LPN/LVN

Long before I was a registered nurse I practiced as a licensed "vocational" nurse. Although I never traveled as an LVN/LPN, I remember hearing all the time, "If only you had your RN license." At the time, I was doing just fine as an LVN/LPN. I never had a problem finding a job, I made more money than I did as a nursing assistant, and still had the satisfaction of assisting the elderly.

That was ten years ago, and I still don't think things have changed that much for LVN/LPNs. You still have LVN/LPNs who are happy to be just who they are and who don't want the added stresses of being a registered nurse. To tell you the truth, there are some days when I wish that I was "only" an LVN/LPN. I still believe that the LVN/LPN is a great asset to the nursing community.

With all that being said, the real question comes to this: how does being an LVN/LPN affect you as a traveling nurse? Should LVN/LPNs be able to travel? Of course. I've met a lot of them that I would much rather work with than some RNs, but there are some hospitals that are phasing them out. This may elevate the degree of difficulty in finding a travel nursing job, but it *does not* make it impossible. To explore this option for LVN/LPNs, I asked for now traveling LVN/LPNs to answer a few questions. The following is what I found out.

When asked if they felt like LVN/LPNs were being phased out, most believe that no, they were not, and that LVN/LPNs should be able to travel as well as RNs because nurses are needed everywhere. The real trick is to gain a lot of experience and have a willingness to travel to limited areas. One nurse stated, “Being an LPN is a financial move; it covers the bases and as in any structured situation, the higher you get the less scutt work you wish to do. Oddly, many good LPN’s don’t see things the same way. Nursing is about getting away from the bedside, and that is understandable; it can be a horrible place to be, but an LPN knows she /he will always be there, so they take it much more to heart than the “office nurse,” and they are always the last in line for respect. It’s a sad way to make a living.”

At the time of writing this chapter it seems like Platinum Select, Clinical One, Gemini Staffing, Aureus Medical, and American Mobile have the most jobs to offer LVN/LPNs. The jobs are as scattered as rehab jobs for me. I would suggest that you find two or three companies and always keep your file updated so you can be ready to go when there is a job that comes up.

When it comes to reimbursements, the jury is split 50/50. Half of the nurses told me that their compensation was no different than an RNs, and half of the nurses stated that their compensation was a little less. From this I gather that it all depends on what company you travel with. Your travel pay, including your housing stipend, meals and incidentals, should be the same whether you’re an LVN/LPN or an RN. The thing that will be different, as usual, is your regular hourly rate.

When it comes to education, the travel companies do not seem to supply much more than your BLS/ACLS. A few hospitals have offered nurses staff positions in trade for financial reimbursement for additional schooling to get their RN license. Personally, I went to school for my RN through the University of the State of New York/Regents/Excelsior program while practicing as an LVN/LPN instead of having a hospital pay my tuition in trade for two years of service. That is a great option if you really want to further your education, but you do not have to get your RN to be a great travel nurse.

Most LVN/LPNs struggle with finding good assignments and the lies, misrepresentation, lack of respect, and lack of recognition. Other facts that challenge LVN/LPNs are reimbursement issues, and they believe that facilities do not want to put their money on LPN/LVN's.

Some of the rewards of traveling as an LPN/LVN include meeting new people, receiving more pay, traveling to places that are happy to see you, and the occasional recognition. Other LPN/LVNs stated that serving the healthcare community and seeing areas of the United Stated that they have never previously visited is what makes it all worth the while to them.

According to most of the company websites that I visited you must have at least two years of experience, with at least six months of recent hospital experience, and LPN/LVNs in a hospital setting must be IV certified. As with traveling RNs, you will still have to file a work history, background check, mandatory education (Blood borne pathogens, OSHA, Fire, HIPPA, etc...), and your skills checklist.

When it comes down to finding a nursing job, I would try one of the "databases" to find out where the jobs are before talking to an individual company. Listed below are the databases that I found with the most job listings:

1. *Medical Workers Database*—A premier job board for physician, radiology, nursing, pharmacy, and other healthcare jobs with an extensive list for licensed practical/vocational nurses. www.medicalworkers.com
2. *Absolutely Healthcare Database*—Absolutely Health Care and HealthJobsUSA is a USA database of healthcare jobs and medical jobs for all areas of health care employment, including, but not limited to allied healthcare jobs, nursing jobs, and physician jobs. Find hospital jobs, nursing home jobs, home health care jobs, school jobs, and outpatient clinic jobs. www.healthjobsusa.com
3. *Nursing Jobs Org.*—A place where you control your own nurse job search. Search for LPN jobs across the U.S. Post your nursing resume in complete privacy and let employers pitch nursing job offers to you. www.nursingjobs.org

~*~

LPN/LVN Travel Companies

All Health Staffing—A national leader in supplementary healthcare staffing, specializing in travel and temporary-to-permanent placement of nurses and other healthcare professionals in a variety of settings throughout the United States. www.allhealthstaffing.com

Advanced Medical Resources —Dedicated to excellence since 1987. www.advmr.net

Advantage Medical Staffing—Do you wear scrubs? We can help you. www.advantagemedicalstaffing.com

Aureus Medical Group—Aureus Medical is the national leader in full-time and travel nursing jobs, diagnostic imaging, therapy and radiation oncology jobs, employment and staffing. www.aureusmedical.com

AWM Staffing, Inc.—AWM Staffing, Inc. is the leader in quality medical staffing services, and we service our medical facility clients by hiring medical professionals who have demonstrated the highest level of service and professionalism. www.awmstaffing.com

Clinical One—From our network of offices throughout the US and overseas, Clinical One recruits select healthcare professionals for placement in travel, contract, per diem, case management and permanent job opportunities nationwide. www.clinicalone.com

Core Medical Group—Their highly experienced staff works with the country's best hospitals to obtain new LPN jobs daily. www.coremedicalgroup.com/lpn-jobs/

Cornice Inc—Will help you make the right move for personal and professional growth. www.corniceinc.com

Gemini Medical Staffing—A staffing company built on integrity and trust. www.geminimedstaff.com

GreyStone Healthcare Staffing—Staffing for long-term nursing and rehabilitation centers located in Florida, Indiana, and Ohio. www.greystonehcm.com

Juno Healthcare Staffing, Inc.—Juno Healthcare Staffing provides staffing solutions that meet the employment needs of hospitals, nursing homes and other healthcare facilities by offering supplemental staffing of nurses, physical therapist and allied healthcare professionals. It offers temporary, full-time, per diem, and traveling nurse jobs for RNs, LVNs, LPNs, CNAs and PTs. You can search for jobs online or get in touch with their recruiters for personalized service. www.junohealthcare.com

Just In Time Staffing, Inc.—Just in Time Staffing. A leader in the healthcare staffing industry. One of the largest databases for LVNs. www.justintimestaffing.com

Kelly Healthcare Resources—Kelly Healthcare Resources® specializes in providing highly skilled healthcare professionals for the hundreds of positions their clients must fill at any given time. www.kellyhealthcare.com

Medical Staffing Solutions: a temporary staffing agency owned and operated by medical professionals with just one mission: Matching the right opportunities with the right people. Local registry jobs as well as national travel assignments are available. www.mssmedicalstaffing.com

Medi-Lend Nursing Services—Frequently asked questions of registered nurses, licensed practical or vocational nurses, certified nurses assistants, allied healthcare providers, hospital administrators and human resource directors. www.medi-lend.com

Meridian Medical Staffing, Inc.—Offers supplemental staffing solutions to premiere healthcare facilities in all fifty states. www.meridianmedicalstaffing.com

Nurses USA, Inc.—Provides expert solutions to healthcare facilities. www.nursesusainc.com

Platinum Select—Outstanding personal service, superior flexibility and premium solutions to fit your every need. www.platinumselect.org

Preferred Healthcare Staffing—Preferred Healthcare Staffing is a leading travel nurse staffing agency with LVN jobs across the nation. They specialize in helping nurses find their ideal travel assignment, with excellent benefits. www.preferredhealthcare.com

Premier Medical Staffing Services—Founded on delivering quality customer service with a personal approach. www.premier.bz

Radius Healthcare Staffing—Works with hospitals, clinics, and skilled nursing facilities to help provide the best quality candidate for permanent or contract positions. www.radiushealthcarestaffing.com

Rn Network—Travel Nursing Jobs from RN Network, the first company in travel nursing to give you first-day benefits for both LPN and RN travel nurses. www.rnnetwork.com

Signature Healthcare—Healthcare Jobs, Travel Nursing Jobs, Nurse Practitioner Jobs, Jobs for Registered nurses, and nursing assistant jobs. Signature Healthcare is here for all your nurse staffing and recruiting opportunities. www.signaturehealthcarejobs.com

Soliant Healthcare—Soliant has opportunities for LPNs in hospitals, nursing homes, private homes, ASCs, and assisted living facilities. www.soliant.com

Supplemental Healthcare—When quality, service and performance matter, health care professionals turn to Supplemental Health Care first. Placing RNs, LVNs, CNAs, therapists and technicians nationwide with travel contracts, per diem or permanent placement positions. www.supplementalhealthcare.com

The Right Solutions—A select group of travel nurse and allied health staffing agencies which has travel contracts for license practical nurses that are IV-certified in military, veteran, and Indian health services. www.therightsolutions.com

Total Med Staffing—A local healthcare staffing company that recruits, screens, and places qualified professionals in various healthcare organizations. www.totalmedstaffing.com

Valley Healthcare Systems Inc.—They understand the value of what their nurses provide and the needs of facilities to have a top-notch staff in an industry that is changing rapidly. It is their commitment to both parties that makes them second to none. www2.vhcsystems.com

Workway Nursing—Specializes in placing skilled licensed practical and vocational nurses in hospitals and long-term care facilities. www.workwaynursing.com

Traveling as an LPN may be a little more difficult than traveling as a RN, but it *is not* impossible.

Chapter Five

Allied Health Travel

Physical Therapy

Physical therapy is a very rewarding occupation in which you can take an immobile patient and have him up and walking in a relatively short time. As a traveling physical therapist you can travel to acute rehabs, home health, pediatric centers, skilled nursing facilities, sub-acute facilities, and wound care clinics.

Many states now require physical therapists to have a master's degree, and it would be a good idea to have at least two years of experience before hitting the road on a travel assignment.

PhysicalTherapyJobServices.com is a full-service informational website that allows physical therapists easy access to many essential resources when planning for a change in your career path. www.physicaltherapyjobservices.com,

Occupational Therapy

When soldiers from WWI came home they needed help to get back to doing even simple everyday activities of daily living. Their "occupation" was getting back to a normal everyday life as best as they could. To help accomplish this, specially trained people called "occupational therapists" were trained to help them get back to the simple tasks of combing their hair, putting on their boots, and feeding themselves.

Occupational therapy has come a long was since then. Now you can not only help those who need assistance at home, on the job or in school, but you can do that for several types of people in several locations around the United States.

In order to be a traveling occupational therapist you will need to be a certified occupational therapy and have at least two year's worth of experience at a hospital or rehabilitation facility.

Speech Therapy

A speech pathologist doesn't just deal with how well you speak, what dialect you speak, or mispronounced words; they are must more than that. They find themselves working in acute care, long-term care, and rehabilitation facilities with those patients who are having problems eating and swallowing. Others also work with patients in improving their linguistics, communication, language disorders, phonetics, and language development.

After completing a "swallow evaluation," speech therapists will make a recommendation on what type of food the patient can handle, whether is whole, cut, soft, ground, or pureed. A speech pathologist or therapists may also accompany a patient to radiology for a barium-swallow test.

Respiratory Therapy

According to the Department of Labor, faster-than-average employment growth is projected for respiratory therapists. Job opportunities should be very good, especially for respiratory therapists with cardiopulmonary care skills or experience working with infants.

The employment of respiratory therapists is expected to grow 19% from 2006 to 2016, faster than the average for all occupations. The increasing demand will come from substantial growth in the middle-aged and elderly population—a development that will heighten the incidence of cardiopulmonary disease. Growth in demand also will result from the expanding role of respiratory therapists in case management, disease prevention, emergency care, and the early detection of pulmonary disorders.

Older Americans suffer most from respiratory ailments and cardiopulmonary diseases such as pneumonia, chronic bronchitis, emphysema, and heart disease. As their numbers increase, the need for respiratory therapists is expected to increase as well. In addition, advances in inhalable medications and in the treatment of lung transplant patients, heart attack and accident victims, and premature infants (many of whom are dependent on a ventilator during part of their treatment) will increase the demand for the services of respiratory care practitioners.

Job prospects. Job opportunities are expected to be very good. The vast majority of job openings will continue to be in hospitals; however, a growing number of openings are expected to be outside of hospitals, especially in home health care services, offices of physicians or other health practitioners, consumer-goods rental firms, or in the employment services industry as a temporary worker in various settings.

Respiratory therapy travel is one field that is gaining in popularity; therefore, the field of traveling respiratory therapy is also growing at an astronomical rate.

For All Therapies

Once you have the license and experience you can travel to hospitals, assisted-living facilities, rehab centers, long-term care center, outpatient clinics, and home health agencies.

Therapists receive some of the same benefits as a traveling nurse, including housing, meals, incidentals, continuing education, free health, dental, and vision insurance along with some short-term, long-term, and life insurance.

~*~

ALLIED HEALTH PLACEMENT COMPANIES

Therapy Jobs—TherapyJobs.com is the leading online resource for physical therapy jobs, occupational therapist jobs and speech therapy jobs. Post your therapy staffing jobs. Therapist, upload your resumé and search jobs for free. www.therapyjobs.com

Advanced Medical Personnel Services—Advanced Medical Personnel Services, Inc. specializes in connecting people with Physical Therapy jobs, Physical Therapy Assistant jobs, Occupational Therapy jobs, Occupational Therapist jobs, and Speech Language Pathologist jobs.

Allied Travel Web—Welcome to AlliedTravelWeb.com, employment site where the search for Allied travel jobs ends. Now travel assignments find the travel therapists, traveling techs and other travel healthcare professionals. Travel companies compete for Allied travelers. www.alliedtravelweb.com

Aureus Medical Staffing—Aureus Medical is the national leader in full-time and travel nursing jobs, diagnostic imaging, therapy and radiation oncology jobs, employment and staffing. www.aureusmedical.com

Bright Med (a division of Temps, Inc.)—BrightMed is the nation's most advanced and innovative employer of health care travelers. Their values are all about trust and building personal relationships that last. www.brightmed.com

Cariant Health Partners—Travel Physical Therapy, Occupational Therapy, and Speech Language Pathology Jobs. www.cariant.com

Comp Health—CompHealth is one of the nation's largest providers of healthcare recruiting and staffing services. www.comphealth.com

Core Medical Staffing—Travel Nursing Jobs. Whether you are seeking a travel nurse, permanent nursing job, or seeking an allied health job, they've got hundreds of health care jobs to choose from. www.coremedicalgroup.com

Cross Country Allied—Cross Country TravCorps offers physical therapy, speech therapy, occupational therapy and respiratory therapy jobs. They also have radiation therapy, speech language pathology, medical lab and other allied health travel positions with thirteen to twenty-six week full-time contracts. www.crosscountryallied.com

Destination Staffing—Traveling physical therapist jobs and occupational therapy opportunities. www.destinationstaffing.com

Foundation Rehab Staffing—They are more than just a job recruiter; they are a personal agent for your career. www.foundationrehabstaffing.com

Guardian Healthcare Providers—Offers customized healthcare professional staffing, recruitment, placement and consulting services. www.guardianhealthcare.com

Health Direction—Physical Therapy Jobs at HealthDirection.com. Specializing in physical therapist jobs, physical therapist job descriptions, physical therapy travel jobs and physical therapy job descriptions. www.healthdirection.com

Hospital Support—Their mission is to build a network of highly qualified healthcare professionals dedicated to working with health care institutions to provide quality patient care. www.hospitalsupport.com

Jackson Therapy Partners—Whether you are interested in travel physical therapy jobs, travel speech therapy jobs, or occupational therapy travel jobs, you will enjoy the same benefits as their permanent partners with the added freedom of choosing the location you want to experience next. www.jacksontherapy.com

Liquid Agents—A comprehensive workforce procurement firm for the healthcare industry. They provide clients with qualified candidates, access to talent database, and cost-effective software. They help nurses and allied health professionals find recognition for their contributions. www.liquidagents.com

MASH Allied Health—They specialize in Travel Nurses, Physical Therapist, Occupational Therapist, Rad Techs, ICD9 Coders on a Contract, Travel and Permanent Placement bases. They have been providing superior service to Healthcare facilities and Candidates since 1987 and have the experience and the knowledge to find what you are looking for. www.mashhealthcare.com

Med Staff America—They are the nation's premier physician search and consulting firm, "where administration and physicians come together." They are a full-service, dedicated and result-driven search and consulting group. www.medstaffamerica.com

Medical Employment Directory—They have been considered the midwest's leading medical recruitment team since 1984. Their goal has always been the pursuit of excellence in Health care Recruitment. They have made thousands of full-time placements, and their team of healthcare recruiters stay informed on the current developments in employment law, medical certifications, and licensing requirements. www.med-search.com

Medical Solutions—Travel nursing jobs and travel allied health jobs are found at Medical Solutions, a JCAHO certified travel nurse agency. www.medicalsolutions.com

Med Travelers—Discover travel therapy jobs and medical imaging jobs at MedTravelers.com. They offer temporary assignments in many disciplines for qualified allied health professionals. www.medtravlers.com

O'Grady Peyton—Their Physical Therapy Program can help you secure a rewarding assignment in America. Physical therapy candidates are encouraged to inquire about available opportunities. www.ogradypeyton.com

Onward Healthcare—Find the travel nurse job, per diem nurse job, or allied healthcare job that is right for you at Onward Healthcare. They are committed to providing their employees with outstanding customer service and the highest paying travel nursing assignments and allied health jobs in the industry. www.onwardhealthcare.com

PPR Healthcare—Specializing in travel nursing and therapy. PPR Healthcare Staffing is an industry-leading employment firm. www.pprhealthcare.com

Protouch Healthcare Professionals—They specialize in permanent placement of allied healthcare professional across the nation. www.protouch.com/allied/

Quality Medical Professionals—A firm specializing in providing the link between those seeking healthcare or medical servicing opportunities and those hiring. QMP provides dependable, affordable staffing services to health care facilities in California. www.iqforme.com

Reflectx Staffing—Therapy jobs at ReflectxStaffing. Looking for a therapy job in Physical therapy, Occupational therapy, Speech therapy, or Respiratory therapy, or have positions that need to be filled? Use their staffing resources to fill your therapy needs. www.reflectxstaffing.com

Rehab Options—A rehab-personnel sourcing service for the rehabilitation services field, and they offer free rehabilitation job listings. Physical therapist jobs, physical therapy assistant jobs, physical therapy jobs, occupational therapist jobs, occupational therapy jobs, occupational therapy assistant jobs, speech-language pathologist jobs, speech-language pathology jobs, speech pathologist jobs, speech pathology jobs, and speech therapist jobs are the positions they cater to. www.rehaboptions.com

Richards Healthcare—Physical Therapy Travel Jobs at Richards Healthcare. Specializing in occupational therapy travel jobs, travel therapy jobs, speech-language pathology jobs and physical therapy jobs. www.richardshealthcare.com

Select Tech Medical—A professional medical recruiting firm that delivers strategic solutions, developing partnerships with their clients, candidates and communities. www.searchtechmedical.com/ancillary.html

Soliant Healthcare—Soliant therapists enjoy excellent salaries, robust healthcare benefits, paid housing and travel, saving plans and much more. www.soliant.com

Special Communication—A therapy groups working in Florida since 1983. Although they do quite a bit of home-based therapy with developmentally-disabled adults, they mostly work at schools, developmental disabilty and early intervention centers. www.specialcommunications.com

Staff Connection—Temporary medical staffing and permanent placement for the health care and medical industry in Michigan and Ohio. www.staffconnections.com

Sunbelt Staffing—They take pride in successfully pairing you with first-rate facilities nationwide. Their commitment to serving you with warmth and having a real interest in your happiness is what makes them different. www.sunbeltstaffing.com

Supplemental Healthcare—When quality, service and performance matter, health care professionals turn to Supplemental Health Care first. Placing RNs, LVNs, CNAs, therapists and technicians nationwide with travel contracts, per diem or permanent placement positions. www.supplementalhealthcare.com

Trustaff—Placing healthcare professionals in travel nurse jobs, pharmacy jobs, therapy jobs, and more. www.trustaff.com

Trillium Healthcare—Focuses on clinical and non-clinical management and medical professional recruitment in the health care sector. Trillium provides a full-service, comprehensive and global approach to health care management and other medical professional permanent recruiting. www.trilliumhr.com

Worldwide Net—A temporary travel healthcare search & placement firm with a proven record of success in the placement of Traveling Healthcare Professionals such as traveling Nurses, CSTs, ORTs, and Respiratory Therapists. www.worldwide-net.cc

Chapter Six

Traveling When You're "Not From Here"

Just because you were not born in the United States does not mean that you cannot become a traveling nurse in the United States. It does take a while to get your work visa, take language tests, take a registered nurse competency test, and make the voyage to the United States, but it is a worthwhile journey when you think about all of the new adventures you will be experiencing. Being a traveling nurse once you have at least one year of experience will give you an excellent way to travel around the United States and see all the wonderful sites. This chapter was written to help you accomplish that dream.

Finding a Nursing Job In United States

With the nursing shortage getting bigger and bigger every day, finding a nursing job in the United States is easier than ever. Nurses who are from the Philippines, Canada, Australia or England can easily gain employment in the United States by following this simple guide.

With the help of CGFNS (The Commission on Graduates of Foreign Nursing School), nurse's qualifications are acknowledged, confirmed and proven in reference to the education, registration, and licensure of nurses worldwide. Through this commission you will need to finalize a Visa Assessment and Work Screen.

In the Work Visa Screen, an educational investigation and evaluation of the foreign nursing license is conducted. Nurses are also required to pass the NCLEX or the CGFNS International Qualifying Examination and an English Language test, such as the TOEFL, IELTS, or TOEIC.

One of the first requirements is getting an associate's or bachelor's degree in nursing and then passing the NCLEX (National Council Licensure Examination), which is a computer nursing competency test.

In some states, if you did not go to an English-speaking school, you will have to take the TOEFL (Test Of English as a Foreign Language) before you can receive your license as a Registered Nurse. This is the most widely used test for workers from a foreign country.

Some states are starting to use the IELTS (International English Language Testing System). It is a language test that measures the ability to communicate in English in listening, reading, writing, and speaking.

The TOEIC (Test of English for International Communication) is an English aptitude examination used as a standard for creating workplace English writing ability and spoken English skills for those who have English as a second language.

After passing the NCLEX, a language test, and obtaining a Visa Screen Certificate you are qualified to submit an application for a nursing license in the state where you reside. Then the fun begins in finding a nursing job.

You would be surprised how many travel companies now welcome foreign educated nurses with open arms. Some of the companies that will assist you include All About Staffing, Assignment America, Global Healthcare Group, Health Careers of America, Nurse Immigration Services, Pacific Link Healthcare, PPR Healthcare, Preferred Healthcare Staffing, Premier Healthcare Professionals, and Worldwide Resource Network.

After visiting these websites, make a short list of which three to five you think will be able to supply your needs the best and then contact them via email. The great thing about these companies is that they specialize in nurses from the Philippines and they can help you every step of the way.

Coming to work in the United States can be a longer process than you would like, but it is important to keep your eye on the cloud with the silver lining ahead of you. Some day, *it will* all be worth it!

CGFNS

The Commission on Graduate of Foreign Nursing, also known as the CGFNS, is a not-for-profit educational organization that evaluates the credentials and authenticates the education of nurses and allied health professionals using their Visa Screen Program.

The CGFNS is dedicated to the registration and licensure of all overseas nurses, whether they are from English speaking countries or not. In order for nurses to obtain their credentials they must take the NCLEX (National Council of Licensing's Exam) and pass an English language test.

The English language tests that you may take include the TOEFL (Test of English as a Foreign Language), TOEIC (Test of English for International Communications), or IELTS (International English Language Testing System). One of these exams must be completed if your education and textbooks were not printed or spoken in the English Language

After you have pass the NCLEX and one of the English language tests the CGFNS will review your Visa Application, and if acceptable, will issue you a Work Visa Screen. To obtain this screen you must also visit the consular officer and inform him/her of your intentions to work in the United States.

To do all of this you must also have a Visa Sponsor, which is a travel company that will assist you in obtaining all the requirements for your Work Visa. Usually this will be attached to you during the time that you work for that travel company.

Work Visa Screen

The Visa Screen is an official document that you will receive from the CGFNS that states that you meet all the legal requirements to work inside the United States and that you are an RN (Registered Nurse). This means that your educational credentials and your competency testing meet the standards for all nurses who wish to obtain a job. The Visa Screen also certifies that you have met the standards set by the Department of Homeland Security.

This screen will certify that you have taken and passed a language test such as the TOEFL, TOEIC, or the IELTS, as described in the section above.

For the VisaScreen you will need to have a license for registered nursing that is not restricted, transcripts from your nursing program showing that you have passed the national council of nursing's licensing exam and obtained a sponsor.

It is also important to note that if you wish to become a resident of New York, Illinois, Florida, Michigan, or Georgia and you have a legal and clear nursing license you may be able to obtain a CGFNS certificate in lieu of the VisaScreen. Related to the nursing shortage, the Department of Homeland security is making it easier for nurses who have a nursing license in another country to get a United States license and this has shortened some of the processes necessary for immigration.

One thing to remember in this process is that there are only limited amounts of Work Screen Visas that are processed every year. The selection is based on the country in which you were born; therefore, going to nursing school in the United States under a student visa does not always guarantee you a work visa.

It is estimated that it will take four months to get a Visa Screen Certificate. You can apply for it at any time and complete all the documents within a year. This means that if you applied on June 30th, you would have until the next June 30th to get in your NCLEX results and your IELTS results, along with all education verification documentation.

After all of this is completed you are on your way to getting a great job as a registered nurse in the United States. And remember that after you get a year's worth of experience you are will have many opportunities to travel and work as a traveling nurse all over the United States. There is no better way to have a career and work at the same time!

English Language Testing

When you make application for your work visa, one of the things they will want to know if you did not go to a school with English textbooks is if you are proficient in the English language. This is accomplished by taking either the IELTS, TOEIC, or TOEFL test. This is a must before you can get a job as a registered nurse.

IELTS stands for "International English Language Testing System." It is a test of English language proficiency. It is jointly managed by the University of Cambridge ESOL Examinations, the British Council and IDP Education Australia, and was established in 1989. There are two versions of this test: the Academic Version (which nurses and medical professionals must pass), and a General Training Version that is used by more than 2,000 universities in the United States.

The IELTS incorporates a variety of accents and writing styles that are presented in text materials in order to minimize linguistic bias. The IELTS tests the ability to listen, read, write, and speak the English Language. Each candidate is scored in four modules: Listening, Reading, Writing and speaking. It is scored on a scale from 1 to 9 with a "9" being an expert user. All nurses must score a total of at least 7, which is classified as a "Good User," which means that he or she has an operational command of the language, though with occasional inaccuracies, inappropriateness and misunderstandings in some situations, and that he or she generally handles complex language well and understands detailed reasoning.

The TOEFL (Test of English as a Foreign Language) evalutes the potential success of an individual to use and understand Standard American English at a college level. It is required for non-native applicants at many English-speaking colleges and universities. Additionally, institutions such as government agencies, businesses, or scholarship programs may require this test. A TOEFL score is valid for two years and then is deleted from the official database. Colleges and universities usually consider only the most recent TOEFL score.

The Internet-Based Test was introduced in late 2005 and has progressively replaced both the computer-based test and the paper-based tests. The IBT is now in use in the United States, Canada, France, Germany, and Italy.

Although the demand for test seats was very high and candidates had to wait for months, it is now possible to take the test within one to four weeks in most countries. The four-hour test consists of four sections, each measuring mainly one of the basic language skills (although some tasks may require multiple skills), focusing on language used in an academic, higher education environment. Note taking is allowed during the iBT. The test cannot be taken more than once a week.

The reading section consists of 3–5 long passages and questions about the passages. The passages are on academic topics; they are the kind of material that might be found in an undergraduate university textbook. Students answer questions about main ideas, details, inferences, sentence restatements, sentence insertion, vocabulary, function and overall ideas. New types of questions in the iBT require paraphrasing, filling out tables, or completing summaries. Generally, prior knowledge of the subject under discussion is not necessary to come to the correct answer, though a prior knowledge may help.

The listening section consists of six long passages and questions about the passages. The passages consist of two student conversations and four academic lectures or discussions. The questions ask the students to determine main ideas, details, function, stance, inferences, and overall organization.

The speaking section consists of six tasks, two independent tasks and four integrated tasks. In the two independent tasks students must answer opinion questions about some aspect of academic life. In two integrated reading, listening, and speaking tasks students must read a passage, listen to a passage, and speak about how the ideas in the two passages are related. In two integrated listening and speaking tasks students must listen to long passages and then summarize and offer opinions on the information in the passages. Test takers are expected to convey information, explain ideas, and defend opinions clearly, coherently, and accurately.

The Writing Section consists of two tasks, one integrated task and one independent task. In the integrated task students must read an academic passage, listen to an academic passage, and write about how the ideas in the two passages are related. In the independent task students must write a personal essay.

It should be noted that at least one of the sections of the test will include extra, uncounted material. Educational Testing Service includes extra material to try it out for future tests. If the test taker is given a longer section he must work hard on all of the materials because he does not know which material counts and which material is extra. For example, if there are four reading passages instead of three, three of the passages will count and one of the passages will not be counted. It is possible that the uncounted passage could be any of the four passages.

The paper-based test is given in areas where the Internet-based and computer-based tests are not available. Because test takers cannot register at the testing center on the test date, they must register in advance, using the registration form provided in the Supplemental Paper TOEFL Bulletin. They should register in advance of the given deadlines to ensure a place because the test centers have limited seating and may fill up early. Tests are administered only several times each year.

With the Internet-based test nurses must make a score of 76. The computer based test is scored on a scale from 0 to 300. Each of the four sections is given a total of 30 points, then these are all added together to get the total score. For the computer test you must make 207, and for the written you must make a 540.

The Test of English for International Communication (TOEIC) measures the ability of non-native English-speaking examinees to use English in everyday workplace activities. It is a two-hour multiple-choice test, consisting of 200 questions divided into 100 questions each in listening comprehension and reading comprehension. Each candidate receives independent scores for written and oral comprehension on a scale from 5 to 495 points. The total score adds up to a scale from 10 to 990 points. The TOEIC certificate exists in five colors, corresponding to achieve results:

orange (10-215), brown (220-465), green (470-725), blue (730-855), and gold (860-990).

The Educational Testing Service (ETS) in the USA developed the TOEIC test based on its academic ETS counterpart, the TOEFL test, following a request from Japan's Keidanren in conjunction with the Ministry of International Trade and Industry, which is today's Ministry of Economy, Trade, and Industry. The ETS's major competitor is Cambridge University, which administers the IELTS, FCE, and CAE.

There were many changes made in 2006, including (1) Overall, passages have become longer; (2) Part 1 has fewer questions involving photo descriptions; (3) The Listening Section hires not only North American English speakers but also British, Australian and New Zealand English speakers. The ratio is 25% each for American, Canadian, British and Australian-New Zealand pronunciation; (4) Part 6 no longer contains the error spotting task, which has been criticized as unrealistic in a corporate environment but instead adopts the task wherein the test taker fills in the blanks in incomplete sentences, and (5) Part 7 contains not only single-passage questions but also double-passage questions wherein the test taker has to read and compare the two related passages such as e-mail correspondence.

Another change in 2007 added speaking and writing tests, and some changes were made to the reading and listening test as well that de-emphasized knowledge of grammatical rules.

This test will take you two hours to complete and consists of 200 questions. Half of the questions are on listening comprehension and the other half is on reading comprehension. Each person receives a score from 5 to 495 on each part, for a total of 10 to 990. Nurses make a score of 725.

After you have completed and passed one of these tests and the NCLEX you can apply to the state board of nursing in which you reside. Through the CGFNS you will then be given your work visa. After you have received your nursing license you are on your way to one year of nursing experience, and then down the road to a travel nursing job.

The NCLEX

The NCLEX is the National Council Licensure Examination which is used to test the competency of all nurses who have completed their required educational program at an accredited university. This test is also required of all foreign-born nurses who wish to come to the United States to practice. This test will be a part of your Work Visa Screen.

This test of 265 questions is performed on a computer. Once you have reached the amount of questions determined by the national council of nursing to prove that you are competent, your test will announce that you have completed the test. Some nurses have gone to 75 and passed, and some nurses have gone to 75 and failed. Some nurses have gone to 265 and passed and some not. Wherever the test shuts off, you really never know how you have done until you get your results in the mail.

The NCLEX-RN (National Council Licensure Examination-Registered Nurse) is a computer-adaptive test (CAT) of entry-level nursing competence. Passing the exam is required of candidates for licensure as a Registered Nurse (RN) by all US state and territorial Boards of Nursing.

The NCLEX-RN and NCLEX-PN examinations are developed and owned by the National Council of State Boards of Nursing, Inc. (NCSBN). NCSBN administers these examinations on behalf of its member boards, which consist of the boards of nursing in the 50 states, the District of Columbia, and four U.S. territories: American Samoa, Guam, Northern Mariana Islands and the Virgin Islands. This test is given only in English.

To ensure public protection, each board of nursing requires a candidate for licensure to pass the appropriate NCLEX examination, NCLEX-RN for registered nurses and the NCLEX-PN for practical/vocational nurses. NCLEX examinations are designed to test the knowledge, skills and abilities essential to the safe and effective practice of nursing at the entry-level.

NCLEX examinations are provided in a computerized adaptive testing (CAT) format and are presently administered by Pearson VUE in their network of Pearson Professional Centers (PPC). Authorized testing centers are located throughout USA and in selected foreign countries, including the most recently approved the Philippines and Mexico. Click on their external link and visit the NCSBN for a list of approved countries where the NCLEX exam is given.

All items are developed and validated, using the expertise of practicing nurses, educators and regulators from throughout the country. The content of the items of the NCLEX examinations is based on a practice analysis conducted every three years. All students considering taking the NCLEX and/or CGFNS exams must keep in mind that the exams are about basic nursing intervention, and not about nursing intervention beyond the level of practice of any entry-level nurse.

The two most important elements when considering and discerning the most correct answer are whether the answer is part of an intervention that is "safe" and "effective." Students should use this as a guideline: if an answer doesn't have the elements of a "safe" and "effective" intervention, whether seeking the physical and/or psycho-social integrity of a patient, that answer cannot be the "best" answer. It can be partially correct, but most likely it is not the best answer of the multiple possible answers.

After you have taken a nursing competency test, English language competency test, obtained a sponsor and have applied for your work visa screen you are well on your way to becoming a travel nursing RN. Once you have that license in hand and work at your sponsored hospital for up to a year you will have the chance to take you skills on the road fulltime with a travel nursing job. Travel nursing RN jobs are not only financially rewarding, but they offer the best way to get around and visit the different parts of the United States.

~*~

Travel Companies Who Assist Foreign Nurses

American Traveler—Travel nurse and travel nurse jobs. American Traveler Staffing offers their travel nurses the highest salaries and best benefits in industry. www.americantraveler.com

Cirrus Medical Staffing—At Cirrus Medical Staffing, they specialize in the placement of traveling medical professionals. If you're ready to earn top dollar, leverage your skills and enjoy the adventure of a lifetime, this is where your journey begins. www.cirrusmedicalstaffing.com

Core Medical Group—CoreMedical Group has been placing healthcare professionals in rewarding travel assignments across the United States. www.coremedicalgroup.com

Expedient Medstaff—A leading travel nurse agency that will bring excitement and adventure to all your future nursing jobs. www.expedientmedstaff.com

Global Healthcare Group—Travel nursing agency with branches and affiliates in the UK, Canada, Philippines, India, South Africa, and the Middle East. www.globalhealthcaregroup.com

Health Staff—Agency that assists qualified registered nurses in preparing for a successful career as a traveling nurse in the United States. www.healthstaffllc.com

Medical Solutions International—A small company that provides quality services to traveling nurses. www.msi-nursestaffing.com

Nurses Rx—Discover the wonderful opportunities NursesRx can provide for Canadian nurses who wish to work in the US. NursesRx is a leading US travel nursing company. www.nursesrx.com

O'Grady Peyton—Learn more about the allied health and nurse employment opportunities at O'Grady Peyton. We offer travel nursing jobs to North American nurses and long-term positions for health care professionals from many other countries. www.ogradypeyton.com

Premier Healthcare Professionals—When you work in the U.S. with PHP, they will assist you with the hassles of relocation so you can focus on enjoying life and practicing your profession. Their dedicated staff will arrange your placement, relocation, housing, and insurance and provide continued support throughout your assignment. www.travelphp.com

Preferred Healthcare—Qualified registered nurses from around the world are in great demand in the United States. Enjoy nursing job opportunities at top hospitals, enjoy great pay and excellent benefits. www.preferredhealthcare.com

Pro Care Nurses—Travel Nurses, Cross country Travel Nursing. ProCare USA is a national healthcare staffing company specializing in placing Registered Nurses and Licensed Practical Nurses on assignments at care facilities throughout the United States. www.procareusa.com

Professional Healthcare Associates—A family-oriented international recruitment firm that specializes in recruiting talented healthcare professionals from all over the world and placing them in the most prestigious hospitals, nursing homes, and medical facilities across the United States. www.phanurses.com

Professional Royal Nurses—A professional healthcare company that provides clinical supervision to independent nursing programs and foreign educated nurses. www.professionalroyalnurses.com

Travel Kare—Providing contract (traveling) and direct staffing of healthcare professionals to hospitals, nursing homes, and home health agencies. www.travelkare.com

Some information obtained through Wikipedia, a public domain governed by a General Public License. For more information, visit their website at: www.wikipedia.org

Chapter Seven

Travel Company Fundamentals

This will be the first major decision that you will have to make after deciding to go on the road full time. There are quite a number of companies out there, and only by understanding the travel company itself, knowing what you want, and doing a lot of research will you be happy in your travel nursing career. There are quite a few that can get you a job, but only a handful that will give you exactly what *you* want.

One of the first things you need to understand about travel nursing is the structure of the agency that you are working for. You may only be in contact on a weekly basis with your recruiter, but people such as the staff supervisor, housing coordinator, payroll specialist, and quality review are some of the others that you will come in contact with.

Recruiter Basics

This is perhaps the most influential person in travel nursing. This is the person in whom you will confide your every want for your career, and who will attempt to give you everything you desire to make you life the fullest that it can be. This is the liaison between you and the hospital. It is their job to help select the appropriate assignment for you. This is the person who takes your profile for a company and submits it to the hospital.

The latest trend in staffing travel-nursing companies is to have the recruiter responsible for bringing in new people, while the staff supervisor is the one who deals with everything "after you're hooked." The staff supervisor then becomes the connection between you and the hospital. Ultimately, you will come to rely on your recruiter or staff supervisor to locate the right obligation for you and ensure that all your needs are being met. This is also the person whom you contact if things are not the way you expected them to be.

One of the advantages of staying with the same company that I have found is that your staff supervisor and/or nursing recruiter will come to know your personality and nursing style. By getting to know you better, what you are, and where you are headed in your travel-nursing career, they can assist you in finding the right path. Remember that your recruiter should be there to assist you at any time. If not himself or herself, then someone should be on-call for the nursing company.

Your recruiter should be an asset to you and your decision and not a hindrance to your nursing experience. Your recruiter should want you to feel comfortable in your new environment. They should be concerned about your safety by not putting you into dangerous situations. Your recruiter should be an asset to you by finding out what you like to do and where you want to go. Your recruiter should know your preferences for a small, moderate, large, or teaching hospital.

This last year I was having a terrible time finding a new assignment, and my recruiter that I have been with for quite a while called me and said, "I know that it is not the location that you really want, but it's close, and I think that you will love the area." Other times she would tell me of jobs, but tell me "I really don't think that you'll be interested in this assignment, but it is available and I just wanted you to know about it." And usually she is right on the money on what I like and where I want to go.

Your recruiter should know your strengths and weaknesses. Just because you are qualified to work on some unit does not mean that you always want to work on that unit. I have approximately five years of rehab nursing, three of telemetry, two of psychiatric, and three years of emergency nursing. I had several companies that refused to find me jobs in any other field besides an emergency room because that was my "specialty," related only to the fact that it was my last permanent position. Hello? I didn't get all that experience just to stay in one field. I got it because I don't want to be told that I can't go somewhere because I'm not "experienced" in what that hospital is looking for.

The Used Car Salesman

Any recruiter, any person, can "sell" you, but do you really want a recruiter or a "used car salesman"? To prove my point, I did some research on what makes a successful car salesman. After visiting just a few websites on the characteristics of a good car salesman, I was astonished at how much the recruiters that I have met had these same qualities.

A recruiter must be personable. What do I mean by "personable"? They must be pleasant in appearance and personality. No, you probably will never *see* your recruiter, but what about their telephone appearance? Good telephone skills are a must with any recruiter. They must have a pleasant voice, and be someone that you *want* to talk to, not someone that you *have* to talk to.

A recruiter must be knowledgeable. It is not a crime not to know the answer to your question, but your recruiter must know where to find the answer. In some research on travel-nursing companies that I have done, several times I was referred to the human resources director, who promptly answered my questions about benefits.

How much does your recruiter know about the nursing field? He might be able to sell you a car, but does he know more about an oil change or a blood transfusion? I am a nurse because I care about people. I want to help others in their time of need and to help them feel better. Sure, I could give someone blood, but what kind of ethics would I have if I just gave the person any old blood without double checking the patient's blood type and double checking the name band before giving that patient the blood? It is a lot easier to replace the oil in your car than to fix a mistake with a blood transfusion.

I'm not saying that the recruiter has to be a nurse, just that they must have extended knowledge of the nursing field. How can a recruiter help you out when/if you get into a bind if they can't understand what is happening at the time? I just don't see how a recruiter can "go to bat" for you if they don't know what they are talking about. These hospitals are hiring travelers because they are short-staffed. Under these conditions, several things can go wrong. I would absolutely refuse to take a position if I didn't feel like I had support from my recruiter.

They must know their product, as well as that of the competition. In order to acquire new nurses, you have to offer the nurse something better than the other companies do. The only way you can do that is if you know what the other companies are offering. Little things, like just a few more dollars an hour or better insurance benefits, can make a big difference. So what if every assignment has a completion bonus if you are making only $20/hour? Attempt to find out what other companies are giving their employees at the same or a nearby location, and then make the deal just a little sweeter, which brings me to my next point of knowing your "customer."

The first thing out of a recruiter's mouth should be, "How can I help you?" So many times, what the recruiter says is translated into, "How can you help us?" These "headhunters" are out there to rope you in no matter what it takes. They *need* you. They don't have a company without the nurse, but so many think that the nurse needs them more. New cars look very nice on the lot, but a lot of good they are doing the salesperson if they stay on the lot.

The recruiter that is going to get my attention is the one that says, "How can I help you fulfill your needs in your nursing career?" Nurses travel for many reasons. The need for a nurse who is fighting bankruptcy is so much different from the nurse who just bought a new car and has a burning desire to see the world.

Above all, a recruiter must have a great personality. I have yet to see a rude, crude, and socially unacceptable nursing recruiter have very many nurses who work for them. Yes, there are some out there, and unfortunately, some of the nurses that I network with have had to work with them, but I have yet to meet a person who will stay with a recruiter who is always on the down and depressed side.

A great personality also means a nursing recruiter who is not only concerned about the benefits of having you work for them, but also what is in your best interest. Like the company that I work for presently—everyone shares the benefits of the nurses; there is no "fighting" for nurses because of that great commission.

A great personality also means that they will be there for you when you need someone to lean on. When the tough times come, you should be able to pick up the phone and discuss the problems you are having with your recruiter. We aren't going to get along with everyone, and not everything is going to be perfect. I want a recruiter whom I can call and tell that I really don't feel comfortable in my current situation because of even such a simple thing as a personality conflict. I want a recruiter who will weather the storm with me, not jump ship and let me feel like I have been stranded in the middle of the desert, begging for water.

The Housing Coordinator

After you have selected an assignment, you will then work closely with the housing coordinator. Their job is to make someplace your home away from home. Most travel companies have contracts with hotels, suites, and apartment complexes in which you get housing paid for by the company. Housing can include or exclude a roommate, selected by you and/or the company. Most companies pay for up to a one-bedroom apartment. A few of the companies even pay for bigger places for your entire family. And yes, the companies encourage your immediate family to travel with you. A happy traveler is a great worker! The company provides all of this for you, although sometimes you might have to ask for it.

If you already have a place to stay, most companies offer a housing stipend in which they give you a certain amount of money that you can use to provide your own housing. These housing stipends are usually tax-deductible, as long as you use the money for business housing. If you take the stipend as a "payroll addition," then it is taxed at the same rate as your paycheck. Many nurses take the stipend and either live with relatives or use it to live in a recreational vehicle.

Housing coordinators make every attempt to find the best housing available for the amount of money that they are budgeted for, according to the bill rate and the housing rate for the area. It frustrates them when something doesn't work out right or they just are not able to provide every stipulation the nurse wants and then all the nurse wants to do is complain about the housing that they did find. Nurses need to realize that it is sometimes very hard to find exactly what the nurse wants at a price that he or she wants.

When I asked housing coordinator Nikki about what makes her job all worthwhile, she replied, "I love finding new housing options that are so awesome I can't believe it. I am such a dork. LOL. I absolutely love my job and almost everything about it. My job always keeps me busy. I don't just find housing; I set it *al l* up for over 200 nurses and handle everything until after they move out."

The Payroll Specialist

A payroll specialist is responsible to make sure that you are paid every pay period. Most companies make this easier by implementing direct deposit. The money is "zapped" from your travel nursing company right into your personal checking or savings account. Although it is your payroll's, or the recruiter's job to put the data into the computer for you to be paid, the payroll specialist is the one responsible for making sure that you get your check in the appropriate time that you are scheduled to be paid. Check with your recruiter or staff supervisor to see who you will turn to if there is a problem with payroll. Some companies prefer you to deal directly with the staff supervisor and some will have you deal directly with the payroll specialist.

Benefits Specialist

You might also come into contact with the benefits specialist. These wonderful people assist you with your benefits from 401K plans, insurance, incentive programs, completion bonuses, and reward programs. Don't be afraid to call them if you think you are not getting all the benefits that you are entitled to. They are very good resources for reliable answers. Unless your recruiter is getting the same benefits as you are, they may not know all the benefits that you are entitled to.

Quality Control Specialist

Some companies even use a quality control specialist, who is like a human resource department that helps you meet compliance criteria for each of your assignments. The quality control manager will help you in all aspects of getting ready for your assignment. I get a call on every assignment from the quality control manager, making sure that my needs are being taken care of by my staff supervisor. In my opinion, this is a *must* for every travel nursing company who wants to have a quality nursing staff. If the nurses are not happy, how can the patients be happy?

Doing Your Shopping

There are plenty of travel companies out there. Do your shopping; do not just grab the first one that makes you an offer. Plan to start looking for a company about a month before planning on going into travel nursing if at all possible. This process will include finding out more about benefits, locations, and general operations of the travel company.

When shopping for a travel company, be aware that some are going to want you to fill out their application and send all of your personal records and qualifications before they will submit you to a hospital. At this point, be careful to give them just your basic information and let them know that you are just shopping for a travel company. Don't make the mistake of filling out applications and checklists for fifty different companies just to interview them.

Also, be careful about who you give your phone number to until you have done your homework. Once you give the travel company your phone number, you will receive phone calls every thirteen weeks, asking you about assignments. It doesn't take long to rack up the minutes on your cell phone.

After reading this chapter, you will be able to find the one company that is going to make you happy in the long run. You will be able to find the one company that goes where you want to go. But first, we need to begin the process of narrowing down your choices.

One thing that should be on that list is your wage requirements. Do you have to have over thirty dollars, thirty-five dollars or can you survive on twenty-five dollars an hour? Know exactly what you need—and not necessarily what you want—to live your new lifestyle.

What kind of housing do you require? If you are single and fancy free? Is motel or extended-stay sufficient? The positives of staying in a motel is that they usually have laundry facilities, a pool, and of course, maid service!

Most companies will provide a one-bedroom furnished apartment. You just bring clothes, linens, and personal items. Watch this option, though, because some companies will tell you that you have a "private" bedroom, when in reality you have a private bedroom with shared common areas with another traveler. This may be fine for a lonely traveler, but most of us like the privacy of our own apartment. This option definitely does not work out if you travel with your family.

Planning to take your family? Most companies will work with you on that. They will provide a two-bedroom apartment for you, although you may be expected to pay utilities or some of the rent.

Another option if you are traveling with your family is to become full-time RVers. This becomes a bit more complicated if you are a female traveler. Not that you can't do it by yourself with a trailer or a 5th wheel, but I would suggest getting a motor home. Motor homes are much easier to move and to park.

As a full-time traveling family, you have the option of your children changing school every three to six months, or you can travel according to the school year. Home schooling is becoming more and more popular and definitely worth looking into. In a later chapter I will discuss the subject of housing and what to do before your first assignment.

What are you location requirements? Do you want to stay in your home state or the surrounding states? With the invention of compact states, you could decide just to travel in compact states. Favorite destinations seem to be Hawaii and Alaska on the west coast in the winter or Maine in the summer, with winter in Florida for the east coast. You might even choose to stay in the middle by going to North Dakota in the summer and to Texas in the winter.

Love to ski? Then go to snow skiing in Colorado in the winter and the lakes of Tennessee for water skiing in the summer. The possibilities are endless.

What about other benefits, such as health insurance, 401K, continuing education requirements, longevity, and completion bonus? These things all matter in your decision!

Find the one company who has the appropriate nursing retention program. What kinds of benefits are added on, the longer that you are with them? Almost all companies have this, whether it is in lieu of money or fits into a reward program.

Don't settle for a company that does not provide a 401K program. Not only should they allow you to put tax-free money in, but they should also be making some kind of vested contribution.

Make sure that the company is reliable. Once you get "out there" in the big world of travel nursing, there are going to be days where the only friend you have is your recruiter or staffing supervisor.

Keep your list handy in your planning stage. As we explore more about your career as a travel nurse, you may want to add more ideas. Don't forget to put on your list the places where you would like to travel. You will need that information because not all travel companies go to all areas of the United States and beyond.

Doing Your Research

Now that you have your list of benefit requirements, use the up-to-date graph, "The Ultimate List Of Travel Companies," on the website http://www.highwayhypodermics.com/ to get an idea of which companies offer the benefits that are most important to you. You will also want to read the chapter in this book entitled "Travel Company Profiles."

Do more research on the Internet by visiting discussion boards and travel nursing forums and ask other nurses what they think of those travel companies. This is where you will find out the inside information on these companies.

Be aware that lurking recruiters may be on the discussion boards and travel nursing forums. Not that I would not talk to them, but just beware that the person who is telling you "Everything is great with this company" might just be working for that company; therefore, you will have a biased opinion.

After narrowing your decision down to about five different companies that you would like to work for, submit a complete application for employment to these five companies.

Upon receiving your application, a recruiter will promptly contact you. Talk to the recruiter and find out what hospitals they have that you are interested in. Find out how many jobs they have available for your specialty. This is especially important if you have a specialty that is on the "hard to find" list, such as psychiatric, rehabilitation, or pediatric emergency care.

Not only should the recruiter interview you, but you should also interview the recruiter! This is easiest done if you get out a notebook to keep track of the questions that you have asked.

Each entry should list the company's name, address, phone number, and the person you talked to. The next entry should be the size of the company. The smaller companies may not have as great a selection of places to travel to, but the customer service is usually impeccable.

Next, you might want to know what kind of structure their recruiters work with. If the recruiters work on a commission basis, you will have a greater chance of a recruiter wanting to sign you up just to make money off of you. If the recruiter is on a shared commission basis you are more likely to find a company that will be based on a teamwork effort, which is always to the advantage of the travel nurse. This also leads to the fact that some companies cater to the hospital, whereas others cater to the nurse.

You will also want to know what the process is in case you decide to change recruiters. When problems arise, you want a recruiter that you feel you can work with. If you feel like the recruiter isn't working hard on your side, or if there are personality clashes, it is much easier to switch recruiters than to switch companies. You don't want to get attached to a company that is not going to work with you on problem solving. Along with this, you also need to find out if there is a recruiter supervisor and who it is. Sometimes this will be the owner in a small company, or a regional supervisor in a larger company.

You will want to know from the recruiter if they can place you regionally, nationally, or internationally. Some companies only cover certain regions, or they have different offices for different regions. Some companies only cover certain states and there are some states that are only contracted with certain companies. If you are interested in traveling internationally, you will want to find a company that specializes in international travel. International travel brings into play a very different set of rules because of immunizations, passports, work visas, etc.

You will want to know how many assignments are available with the company. This is especially important if location is your number one priority. If this requirement isn't fulfilled, then you are going to find yourself hunting for a different company for each assignment.

You will need to find out what kinds of specialties are offered through the company. The most common specialty companies that I have found are companies who specialize only in providing hospital operating room personnel. A few companies out there specialize only in providing management personnel. If your specialty is med-surg, you will have quite a few companies to choose from; but if your specialty is psychiatric or rehabilitation, you might have trouble finding a company who provides those types of jobs.

You need to get out your list of priority benefits and ask about those. Your priority benefit list might include the type of insurance they provide, the name of the company their insurance is with, whether it's a PPO, HMO, or just a major medical plan. What are the deductibles and how much does the insurance cost the travel nurse? Yes, there are companies out there who provide free medical insurance for their travel nurses. This is a question that you have to ask yourself: are you willing to pay a small amount for your insurance?

You will want to know when you will be paid and how you will be paid. Most companies will send you a weekly check, but there are some out there that only pay bi-weekly or monthly. If you receive a housing stipend, find out if you will be paid the stipend on a weekly or monthly basis. Are monthly stipends paid at the first of the month or at the end of the month?

You will need to find out if the company writes guaranteed hours into their contracts. How many hours do you want to work? Some companies will give you a guarantee of thirty-six hours, while others will guarantee you forty-eight hours. Are those hours broken into eight-hour shifts, ten-hour shifts, or twelve-hour shifts?

What length of assignment does the company offer? In a fast response situation, you might find assignments lasting only four weeks. At other places, you might find companies that offer six to nine month contracts. For those nurses who are traveling with school-age children, maybe a nine-month contract during the school year would be preferred over a short-term contract.

If you take the housing, then you will want to know what type of housing is available. Are there are any additional costs to the traveler? Will you have to share housing with another traveler? If you take the subsidy, you will want to know if they pay just what your expenses are, or if you get to keep any of the extra money if there is any left over after paying your expenses. The housing subsidy should be equal to the cost of renting a one-bedroom apartment.

Another thing that you might want to know in the company interview is if airfare and rental car fees are provided. This is especially true if you plan to travel somewhere outside the continental forty-eight states, such as Hawaii, Alaska, or the Virgin Islands. Airfare is definitely needed for a trip to Hawaii, but some travel nurses opt out of the rental car fees and purchase a vehicle from other travel nurses who are leaving the island.

Submission Requirements

What is required before you can be submitted to a hospital? With most companies, all you need is an application for employment, a skills checklist, and a resumé. Other travel companies will want all the ducks in a row before they will even submit you. If you are sure that you want to go with that company and location, then go for it, but be careful about filling out too many forms for too many companies. This can be very time consuming, and in effect, wasting time if you are not serious about working for that company.

After the interview, if you feel comfortable in continuing a relationship with those companies, then fill out the checklist. One mistake I made when I started out was to fill out the checklist and an application with about 30 different companies. Not only did it take several days to do all of those applications and checklists, but my phone wouldn't stop ringing.

Personally, I never give out the phone number of my current place of employment. Some recruiters don't care how busy you are; they are out to secure you—"their" travel nurse—and you have the problem of too many phone calls at your current place of business. And yes, whatever company you are looking at, they do have recruiters that work in the evening and at night!

Once you have decided on a travel company you will need to pick a place for them to submit your profile. Be very careful to keep track of what company has sent your profile to which hospital. Your chances at that hospital can be ruined if two different travel companies submit your profile.

Chapter Eight

From The Other Side

My job as a traveling nurse is to go from hospital to hospital and give patients the best care that I can. Although some people choose the independent contractors route, I personally love to have a great company take care of such things as payroll, taxes, and housing.

I have been to several company offices, and I have some idea what it is like to be on the other side, but to get a better grasp on the reality of things, I asked a few others that are in the trenches to help me get a better look at the company side. The following chapter the information that was supplied to me from people in human resources, housing, payroll, and a lot of recruiters.

I firmly believe that by understanding the other side, a stronger bridge can be built between the travel nurse and the company. After all, we need to act like a team instead of arch- rivals.

~*~

Human Resources

My first interview is with Shirley, a director of administrative services for a national travel nursing company. This is what she had to say about the human resources part of the travel nursing business.

"Benefits were made to be used to offset skyrocketing healthcare costs when you need treatment. That is why our organization pays for our travelers' benefits in full each month. We research various insurance companies yearly to ensure that our travelers are receiving the maximum insurance coverage while containing the cost.

In addition, those who elect to join 401(k) programs need to take the time to read how to manipulate the 401(k) website that's assigned to those who join. You are able to track your investments and returns on a weekly basis, if you choose. Some travelers don't take the time to do their homework. The benefit is clearly to the traveler's advantage, but most don't recognize the value.

As long as our travelers understand that they have the right to ask and have the right to an answer in a timely manner, we're glad to help them in any way possible. Other free benefits including continuing education, online forms, online payroll stubs, vacation pay, earned paid time off days and the like make being a traveler less complicated and risky. Make sure that you're able to use these things to your advantage! If you're not sure, feel free to ask. That's what we're here for!"

Another responsibility of human resources is the hiring of recruiters. It's human resources that take the applications, verify previous employment and set up the interview of the candidate. According to Monica, at Trinity Healthcare Staffing Group, a great recruiter is one that is well spoken, has a great phone voice, good phone skills, and a nice personality. Some recruiters come from such backgrounds as nursing, banking, or retail. Human resources is also responsible for the extensive training that a recruiter must go through after accepting the position.

The recruiter then becomes a human resource for the nurses who want to know about insurance benefits, co-pays, deductibles, how much and when the insurance and 401K comes into effect. Nurses need to know that if their recruiter cannot answer the questions that there usually is an HR person readily available to answer those questions.

~*~

About Payroll

Benefits are wonderful, but we all desire a great paycheck. We work our time and fax our time cards, but if the ball stops there we are very unhappy when our paycheck doesn't arrive. If nursing and payroll work together, things go much smoother and nurses get the correct amount, either weekly or bi-weekly. Imagine walking into an office on Monday morning and having hundreds of faxes, with some even flowing onto the floor, and trying to put everything together.

Tara, a payroll coordinator, tells me that she loves to have travelers not only have their time sheet faxed in on time, but also call their recruiter to make sure that it has been received. Her biggest pet peeve is when nurses write their time on notebook paper rather than the time sheet and do not sign their time sheets. She states, "I love the people and environment that I work in; I just wish that nurses would understand that to pay them correctly, it really helps to have a nice clear time sheet. You would be surprised at the way some of the nurses complete their time sheets. Some are just a mess."

Payroll can be difficult at times, considering the fact that this department is responsible for making sure that the nurse is paid the contracted amount, correct the amount if changed by a contract renewal, making sure that the nurse's time sheets and the kronos or hospital report matches, and keeping track of per diem daily pay. A typical Monday and Tuesday is spent keying the nurses' time into the payroll computer system, with Wednesday used ass a problem-solving day. Thursday is used for invoicing and reimbursements, with Friday used as payday and more problem solving.

A common thing that causes some confusion between the nurse, hospital, and travel company is when the hospital's pay week and the staffing company's pay week do not match. Nurses need to talk to their recruiter or payroll department to find out how to effectively go with the hospital's schedule so the hospital isn't paying for two days on one week and a fourth overtime day on the second week. This can cause a major headache for all involved in this type of situation if it is not handled properly.

Mike has this to say about his job as a payroll controller: "Payroll in the travel nursing industry is extremely complicated. Some have their housing paid, while others receive monthly housing stipends; travel pay is due on different dates; weekly pay includes taxed income, or some elect to receive a portion of their income tax free (tax advantage plan); reimbursements for nursing licenses, other applicable bonuses from time to time; hospitals observe different holidays and different hours to receive holiday pay; notes on timesheets written from travelers are sometimes not legible. You also have to consider the nurse's request for paid time off days and vacation pay. It doesn't appear to be that complicated, but multiply that by several hundred travelers weekly and it becomes very complex!

With this type of complexity, mistakes can occur. It's what your travel company does about the situation and the response time to correct it that makes a difference. We, like everyone else, make mistakes. We create processes and modify processes each time mistakes occur in order to minimize them from reoccurring. We even go as far as to wire it into our traveler's bank accounts immediately, if it's our mistake, at no cost to the traveler. Some of these mistakes can be avoided by getting timesheets in on time. This permits our payroll department to ensure that your pay is correct before meeting the deadlines to be processed by payroll firms and entered into your direct deposit account in time for you to be paid on time."

~*~

Housing Department

The best job at the best hospital can be miserable if you don't have the right housing. This can be really complicated, in that housing coordinators try to make arrangements for housing without ever stepping foot into the housing. Pictures are worth a thousand words, but we all know that pictures are of "the best" apartment in the place, and not necessarily the one that you will be moving into. In today's day and age, most housing arrangements are made from resources found on the Internet.

As stated in a previous chapter, if you find the housing to be absolutely unacceptable, it is your responsibility to let the housing department know as soon as you arrive. Look the apartment over very carefully before moving all your belongings in and accepting the apartment. Do not accept any apartment that is not suitable for human living. Any company that really cares about their travel nurses will offer to put you up in a hotel until proper housing can be found. You do *not* have to live with bedbugs and cockroaches!

Nurses also need to understand that you cannot have Dom Perrion champagne on a Cold Duck budget. Not saying that you can't have champagne, but you have to operate within the limits of your budget.

Housing coordinator, Nikki, states that what she expects from a nurse is just for the nurse to work with her and understand that she is doing everything in her power to supply the greatest housing that she possibly can, within her budget limits.

It just drives her crazy when something doesn't work out right or she is not able to provide every stipulation that the nurse wants, and sometimes they get kind of nasty with her. "There has never been a time when I have not exhausted every possible option to give them exactly what they want." Nurses need to realize that although she always does her absolute best to find what they want, it isn't always possible.

Nurses must understand that not only does the housing coordinator find the apartments, but they set up all the utilities and rental furniture before and after the nurse's assignment. This is not only done for one or two nurses, but for hundreds of nurses.

~*~

Quality Assurance

I recently spent a lovely morning with the quality assurance team for Trinity Healthcare Staffing and found the girls in the office to be quite pleasant. I sincerely hope that after this section of the book, nurses will have a better understanding of the functions of this department, and that they really aren't the "QA nazis" that some nurses have them labeled as. Instead of being defined as "a person who fanatically seeks to control a specific activity or practice," they need to be thought of as a department that is dedicated to assuring that the quality of the nursing staff is well documented.

Their job is one of the toughest in the industry, due to the fact that it is their task is to keep up with what the hospitals have to have as far as immunizations, urine drug screens, medication testing, background checks, and other tests that are required, especially if the company is JCAHO certified.

As I walked into the QA office, I faced a large board with the requirements for several vendor management and hospital associations, through which most travel nursing contracts are processed. Next to each vendor management name was a list of the particular requirements for that state or regional area. No two vendor management companies required the exact same things. Some require only one PPD, while others required two... others required titers for chicken pox, while others required just a statement that you have had the disease.

Before a job can be confirmed, all of the nurse's ducks have to be in a row in this river of paper. It is the quality assurance analyst's job to make sure that the nurse's paperwork is in line for the job that they are going to accept, and if it isn't, then it's their job to make sure that they get it. Therefore, they have to notify the recruiter of things needed to complete the file, and the recruiters have to "bug" the nurses until all the paperwork is in. Although this can be very annoying, nurses have to realize that this is required from the hospital to the nursing staff company.

~*~

From The Recruiters

Not only do I often wonder what my recruiter really looks like, I wonder exactly what they are faced with on a day-to-day basis. Some nurses truly believe that all recruiters do is sit behind a desk and try to talk nurses into an assignment just to fill out their monthly quota sheets or have great wealth related to commissions earned from placing nurses. It is amazing to me that people truly don't realize that we, as nurses, only take care of less than ten patients a shift, but recruiters are responsible for twenty to fifty nurses.

To take a more in-depth look at this side of the business, I set up a survey online and sent an email to all the travel companies that I am in contact with. This is what the recruiters had to say about their side of the business.

~*~

Meg has been a recruiter for one year. Her ideal travel nurse is someone who communicates with her on a regular basis. She likes to stay in contact and make sure both the nurse and the facility are happy. She wants a nurse or therapist who has great clinical skills and is able to get along with others. They should be able to adapt to different work environments.

The most frustrating part of her job is when she has a great nurse and can't find the perfect contract for them, but she loves it when a nurse calls from their assignment and tells her how much they love it and how happy they are.

She is available twenty-four/seven for her nurses. She makes every attempt to develop a personal relationship with all of her nurses, and they are her priority. She is not a sales person; she just tells the upfront truth about assignments and expectations.

~*~

Brie has been a recruiter for two years. What she looks for in a traveling nurse is someone who understands that recruiters are human too. The recruiters are just trying to make their way in the world. It's not likely that the travel company you work for sits around a boardroom, rasping their fingers, thinking of ways to make travelers' lives miserable. We want you to be happy!

The most maddening part of her job is calling or emailing someone and never getting a response. She can take "no" for an answer, but for some reason she can't stop until she hears it. The most gratifying part of her job is when a nurse treats her like a co-worker or teammate.

She would like nurses to know that they can relieve a lot of stress about travel nursing if they give themselves a couple of good options and keep an open mind about locations. Every hospital could probably use a traveler, but there are many hoops to jump through for it to be official. "We're working on it," she promises. Her best advice is, "Have fun, enjoy the country, and don't sweat the small stuff!"

~*~

Pam has been a recruiter for three years. Her ideal nurse is someone who understands that as a recruiter, they are not out to "get them" or rip them off. She is looking for someone who is honest and that is looking into an assignment. What frustrates her the most is when she does all the leg work for a travel nurse and they are not honest enough to tell her "Yes, we are interested" in the assignment or "No, we really are not interested." It is also frustrating when someone accepts an assignment and then doesn't show up. She also would like someone who is not going to complain if the wallpaper in the bathroom apartment doesn't match the wallpaper in the kitchen. Someone who is not afraid to say to say, "I am working with another agency, and they are offering me this. What can you offer me?"

Another frustrating part of her job is when a nurse who is so motivated for an assignment, that you push and push to get all the numbers right, all the documents correct and submitted, get the nurse interviewed, and then the nurse becomes missing in action, or can't make a decision regarding whether they are interested or not.

The most gratifying part of her job is matching a great nurse with a great hospital, and coming to find out that her nurse has found her soul mate in the area of his or her assignment.

She would like other travel nurses to know, "We are all a team; good recruiters want the best nurse to meet the best hospital and it to be a perfect match. We also want nurses to know we know how hard they work; we know of all the crap they go through, and that's why a good recruiter is here to back them up if something goes wrong, or if they are not happy. That's why we are on call twenty-four/seven. We are taking time away from our families to make sure they are taken care of, no matter what."

"Nurses and recruiters have a lot in common; we both take a lot from people who at times don't truly appreciate what we really do."

~*~

Lindsay has been a recruiter for five years and has learned that every nurse is different. She has also found that those who have realistic expectations are flexible, to an extent, but not to the point that they need to change their name to "Gumby." She also has found that a nurse who gives as much as what's given to them makes the best traveler.

What frustrates her the most is working very hard with a new RN, only to find that after an offer is made, or worse, even accepted, they have fallen off the face of the Earth. She states, "I work hard to be up front and honest, and I expect the same from the travelers I work with. If you don't want the assignment or something better has come up, just let me know! I understand that these things will happen, but if there is open communication, things can be resolved in a positive way."

The most gratifying part of her job is when she does go that extra mile for someone and knowing that she has made a positive impact on their lives.

She would like travel nurses to know that not all recruiters are out there to make as much as possible off of their travelers by doing as little as possible. There are definitely some less than ethical recruiters out there, but those that she knows and trust will bend over backwards to make an assignment enjoyable for all parties involved. She has gone to bat countless times for her travelers; whether it is with her higher-ups or a hospital. She is very proud of that fact.

When asked about final comments, Lindsay states, "It's either a good fit for all, or it's not a fit at all."

~*~

Teresa has been a recruiter for five years. She is looking for experienced travelers that can communicate, respect and empathize. As hard as she tries, sometimes she just cannot fix everyone's problems. She loves her nurses, but at times she does feel like a doormat.

The most annoying part of her job is when a nurse walks out on a contract without any remorse.

She really tries the best for her nurses and makes every attempt to give one hundred percent. She looks out for her nurses and prides herself in getting to know her nurses and becoming friends with them. She makes every effort to treat her nurses like family.

"I love my job and my nurse friends I have made over the years. This has been a very rewarding job. I believe that this is what I am supposed to be doing at this point and time of my life."

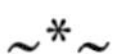

Carol has been a recruiter for five years and looks for someone who is willing to listen to all the information that she has to offer for an assignment before asking, "How much?"

Although she hates the endless calls, it is thrilling to finally reach someone who is willing to talk about an opportunity.

She would like all travelers to know that the recruiter is between a "rock and a hard place" as far as rates go. They are contractually bound to their member hospitals to try to save them as much money as possible, while attempting to give the nurse what they expect in a travel assignment.

Jack has been a recruiter for ten years and looks for someone he can believe in. He wants someone who will partner with him versus just work with or work for him. He likes taking care of people also, so letting him help a traveler out makes him feel good. He looks for nurses who have a good heart and are looking for a friend, not just a recruiter.

What burns him is having to overcome what other recruiters have done to the traveler. It really creates a barrier when a recruiter gives the traveler a raw deal. Breaking down that wall, making the traveler understand that he is not like those others is very difficult and frustrating.

The best part of his job is having a nurse call him when he is lying at home sick during the week just to make sure that he is taking his medication. Jack states, "I have done this for so long that the only thing that makes me feel good is to become a friend to the nurses."

He would like all the nurses to know that not all recruiters are "snakes." There are some recruiters that actually do care and do this type of work for the enjoyment of it. Not all recruiters are sales people, and some of them are honest.

~*~

Greg has been a recruiter for nineteen years and looks for someone who is focused in their career and experiencing various opportunities at both small and large facilities in various locations, someone who wants to expand their location beyond their backyard. He looks for someone who not only represents themselves well, but would represent his company well. Someone who is dedicated enough to work their committed hours fully and comply with paperwork and contractual requirements.

The most aggravating part of his job is getting travelers to get their paperwork in on time, getting them to consider all opportunities instead of one that's one hour from their home, getting their timesheets in on time so as to not cause payroll processing issues with direct deposit, and travelers not working their fully assigned hours. It also doesn't make him happy when travelers don't always do what they say they'll do and think that it's ok for them to ignore the recruiter, but never ok for the recruiter to ignore the traveler, regardless of how faithful the recruiter is to the traveler.

The most rewarding part of his job is seeing travelers blossom into worldly individuals who not only understand healthcare, but also the business of healthcare, witnessing their successes, developing the personal relationships over long periods of time, and getting them the job that they want.

The following is Greg's insight to the world of travel nursing. "I like all of our travelers, but cannot take one hour to talk to each of them daily. No one at my firm is trying to rip them off, regardless of their history with other firms; we're not trying to "pull the wool over anyone's eyes". You don't have to scream, threaten to walk, threaten legal action, or report to whatever agency in the sky that will close us down. Just tell us the issue and trust us to do our job and follow through. That means it usually can't be fixed in ten minutes. You have to give us time to correct what's wrong. Making demands of your recruiter will net you nothing. The more demands, the less attractive the traveler becomes. We bend over backwards to get you what you want, so if we get it for you, we expect you to take what you've committed to take. Travelers who are open to go most places are the ones who make more money and are more fulfilled with their careers. It is great to compare firms, but compare apples to apples. If one firm offers paid insurance and the other benefits stink, why keep penalizing the firm with the bonafide good benefits for more money when the firm already takes care of their travelers from the get-go? If benefits are your cup of tea, then get with a firm with good benefits. If not, go for the cash with another firm."

Out of all the travelers that Greg has met in the past nineteen years, there has been only a handful that he would absolutely refuse to work with. "All in all, travel nurses are a great group of talented professionals!"

Concerning the financial aspects of a travel company, Greg states, "Containing overhead costs while giving travelers what they're asking for is a true juggling act. We try to do everything possible to meet travelers' expectation while providing top pay, benefits and perks, yet we have to maintain a financially stable organization that provides security, support and appropriate staffing levels to our travelers. When a traveler walks out on a contract without giving notice or doesn't show for an assignment, the investments that we've made prior to their start date is lost money related to a three-month apartment lease, furniture delivery costs, furniture rentals, utility setup, etc. Those costs add up over the period of a year. We could have given that money back to our other travelers, purchased another benefit or enhanced something for the rest of our travelers. These types of actions damage the reputations of travelers at facilities and isn't fair to the travelers who take their commitments more seriously."

~*~

Nikole has been a recruiter for four years, and her ideal travel nurse is someone who is knowledgeable about the industry and what is realistic. She receives a lot of requests that are difficult, and sometimes even impossible to place. For example, a very common request is a barely two year med-surg nurse demanding to make $40 per hour, usually in a state such as Hawaii. The industry has definitely changed from only a few years ago and most nurses she speaks with are not aware of how he/she is actually compensated for a certain area. Basically, she would like to deal with professionals that are honest with good work ethics.

The most frustrating part of her job is that the competition aspect can be extremely overwhelming. Her company is constantly being compared to what this or that company is offering, so it seems like she is always bidding with other companies. Usually, the company with the best monetary offer wins every time. It doesn't seem that honesty and hard work takes you very far some days.

The most enjoyable part of her job is the great feeling she gets when she is able to make a placement and the nurse enjoys the housing and the facility. It's very rare that everything comes together perfectly, so it is a wonderful feeling of accomplishment when it does.

She would like travel nurses to read books, magazines and forums that explain where the industry is at this point and try to understand how things really work in this business. She would also like them to know that as a recruiter, there is a very negative impact when a nurse jeopardizes a contract or simply decides it's not working, without any attempt for improvement. The recruiter often absorbs the cost of apartment leases broken, etc. She has done both recruiting and nursing, and in no way is one harder than the other. They are both extremely difficult jobs that require a lot of commitment, and the recruiter is not necessarily profiting largely off of the nurse's hours worked.

When told about this chapter, Nikole stated, "I think that this is an awesome way to learn about the healthcare travel industry...for both travelers and recruiters."

~*~

Kim has been a recruiter for fifteen years, and to her the ideal travel nurse is a person that is open-minded and willing to team play with their recruiter. There are so many different facets of travel. A nurse has to be willing to be a flexible person, with an attitude that makes them desired for a contract to be extended. Attitude is 85% of a good traveler. Rules are important, but we are always ready to listen to all sides of a story.

The most infuriating part of her job is trying to accommodate all the personal needs and emergencies that come to light each and every day. It also makes her cringe to have a traveler tell her they must go somewhere, and then take a job in a completely different state and different pay rate than requested. Travelers who make a commitment for a job and then back out also drives her crazy, as well as not showing up for the assignment and not talking to her.

The most rewarding part of her job is seeing a nurse get to their destination and everything to be just as stated. She also enjoys hearing a nurse tell her for the first time that their bills are caught up and being told that the traveler got to see their family for the first time in years. Kim takes pride is making sure that all problems are resolved in a timely fashion, and it's always nice to be told when the nurse appreciates her. The most satisfying part of her job is being told that she has made someone's dream come true.

She would like travelers to know that there are so many things to learn about before one travels. Expectations are high for a travel nurse, and it's not for everyone. It is important to know that you have a great relationship with your recruiter, as they will be your main connection to all problem resolutions. Make sure that you feel great about the company, the contract and the person that you have that one-to-one relationship with—the recruiter. This is a great journey and experience; make this commitment and keep it.

"When one decides to travel, they should do lots of research and ask many questions. It's a major decision for you, or even your family. Gain as much information as possible about the company that you choose and ask questions of the recruiter. Get to know them on a personal basis and make sure that they are as committed to working for you as you are for them. This is like a business partnership, and you have to have a support system. Make sure you feel great about every aspect of your journey."

~*~

Jenny has been a recruiter for two years, and her ideal travel nurse is someone who is experienced and well skilled in several different modalities, giving them the ability to float. Travelers are also expected to hit the floor running; therefore, she prefers someone who can walk into any hospital and get to work. Flexibility is also very important; they must be flexible with their shift, schedule, and geography. Other qualities of a great travel nurse include someone who has great people skills, interacts well with patients and staff, and who acts like a professional, someone who is responsive and responsible, updates information upon request, turns in their timecard in a timely manner, and someone whom you trust and are proud to have working for you. Most importantly, a nurse who is a nurse because they love it—they love taking care of people.

The most frustrating part of the job is working with nurses who have unrealistic expectations, and losing great nurses.

The most gratifying part of the job is being able to help out hospitals that are short staffed, the better staffed they are, the better care patients get. It's also fun to work with so many different people from all over the country and to hear all their adventures. It's great when you hear a nurse say "I love my assignment."

She would like nurses to know that as recruiters, they do everything they possibly can for them—financially, geographically, and with the hospital—but you have to understand that they have guidelines and rules they have to follow as well. Recruiters are here to help; they are an advocate of the nurses. All they ask is that you are flexible and patient; they are doing everything they can. She would also like nurses to know that this is a job; recruiters take it very seriously and nurses are expected to do the same. Nurses are required to show up for work on time as scheduled, are responsible for making sure that everything that is required of them by both the company and the hospital is in and completed, including their timecards. Nurses represent the company they work for and they are expected to act as professionals, just as they expect the company to do.

~*~

Jessica has been a recruiter for over six years and states that she looks for a nurse who is still a nurse because he/she loves what they do—help and heal. She also looks for a nurse who exhibits some flexibility. She understands that nurses are very proud of their accomplishments and their advancements through their field, and they respect, honor and even celebrate that, but when an intensive care nurse refuses to float to telemetry or med/surg or the emergency room because they think it is beneath them, the only ones who suffer are the patients, due to the ego of another human being.

The most annoying part of her job is the fact that some nurses don't feel that they can be honest with them about their true level of interest in going to a certain location. She hates going through the hassle of getting paperwork and getting them submitted somewhere in New York City, only to find out that the nurse really wanted to be in Florida, just as an example.

It warms her heart when she places a nurse on an assignment and she thinks about all the people that the RN is going to touch in their short thirteen weeks that she is going to be there, related to the fact that she is not a nurse or has the capability or emotional strength to get out there and treat people as a nurse does. She feels like she has really made a difference in those people's lives as well. Just by finding that stellar RN who loves her job gives her great satisfaction and keeps her going.

The three things that she would like nurses to know the most are the following: (1) There are a number of companies out there that don't hire their recruiters on a commission basis; (2) Recruiters understand that the pre-employment paperwork is a real hassle, but in order for us to do a service to our facilities we need to be compliant on our side; (3) And recruiters love their jobs and are doing this because they enjoy helping people also.

~*~

Millie has been a recruiter for four years and prefers a nurse who communicates with her. She believes that it helps to make the assignment a good one. She needs to know exactly what the old- timers and newbies require to make the assignment not only a good one, but a great one. Not every assignment is a perfect match, but she will do as much as possible to make it livable for thirteen weeks. It is important to know the location that the nurse desires, the pay, the benefits, the housing, and if there is any family or pets traveling. Tell her what you need to make it work, and don't forget to return her calls.

It is also important for her to know when you get a call from the hospital that you have been submitted to, and to know if your plans change. If there are several agencies trying to get an assignment for you, let her know that also, to prevent double submitting you to a hospital. The best recruiter and nurse relationships are built on trust and communication. It is very important to keep in touch, even when not on assignment to maintain connections for the next road trip together. Other characteristics that Millie desires most in a nurse are integrity, honesty, friendliness, professionalism, a desire for adventure, and flexibility.

The most frustrating part of her job is not having the right spot at the right time for someone. She can have twenty emergency room needs and no one ready to go. When she has to have that need and it's not there, it's very frustrating. Not having the money that everyone is worth isn't easy either. It is also aggravating when someone does not call her back after she has searched the orders daily for their specific need. It is all in divine timing!

The most satisfying part of her job is when an assignment works for the nurse, family and the facility. It is music to her ears when she hears "*I love* this assignment." She also enjoys the friendships that develop through the journey, from the first call to the decision to settle down...it makes it all worthwhile.

When asked what she really would like nurses to know, she states, "I love what I do... I come from a rural area in upstate New York. I have traveled and lived in different areas of the United States. Some of the places I liked, other places, well... you made your own fun. I know what its like to be away from family. I have an adventurous spirit and joined the Navy to do my part for my country during the Vietnam War in 1973-79. I believe we all should be able to go where we want to go, live where we want to live, and have the freedom to do what we want to do. I am happy to do my part to keep all the adventurous travelers traveling."

~*~

I received an email that really sums up the aspect of being between a rock and a hard place in an effort to please both the hospital and the travel nurse.

Jeff, a vice president of nursing recruitment, states that his company goes through painstaking measures to ensure contractual compliance with their travelers, and he expects them to live up to their contractual commitment as well. He does not, however, expect them to be a doormat to any client or agency. He needs to know of working issues immediately so he can spearhead a win/win resolution. Other than that, he appreciates mutual respect.

Jeff and his crew all agree that they love making their travelers happy and building lasting relationships. They also agree that they become very protective of those travelers whom they have come to know and trust.

It absolutely drives him crazy when issues surface related to the fact that paperwork is not completed on time. Recruiters understand that travelers might have been treated poorly by some agency, somewhere, sometime; however, that has never (nor will ever) be our intent. Just keep "your head on," tell us your issue, and you'll be amazed of the lengths to which we'll go to resolve an issue quickly and fairly.

Travelers also need to understand that hospitals constantly cancel contracts when the proper documentation isn't in place prior to an assignment. Hospital human resource departments set tight deadlines to get paperwork to the hospital prior to the start of the traveler's assignment. All firms have to deal with issues regarding traveler and client dissatisfaction. What's important is the speed and accuracy of correcting the issues satisfactorily and ensuring a smooth start for the traveler for each assignment.

Jeff would like nurses to know that they always include their input in their plans to enhance what their company does for their travelers. Whether they're a difficult personality or not, recruiters want travelers to be fulfilled by what they do, how they support them, and how they are treated. "We respect each of our travelers for who they are and for their role with patients, patient families and their clinical talents. Because of this, we will always protect their best interests. We know who 'butters our bread' and our employees are reminded daily."

~*~

A big thanks to all the recruiters and companies who made this chapter possible, including Across America Med Staffing, Adex Medical Staffing, Aureus Nursing, Cirrus Medical Staffing, Integrated Nursing Alliance, Nursing Innovations, RN Demand, Response One, and especially to Trinity Healthcare Staffing Group, who allowed me to spend two days hanging out at the office and ask questions of the staff there, which has allowed me to have an even more in-depth look at what it really is to be on the other side at the staffing office.

Chapter Nine

Location, Corporation, and Documentation

Just where would you like to start your travel nursing career? There are a lot of choices! You can choose a large teaching hospital in a metro area, a small hospital in a big city, a big hospital in a smaller town, or a small town with a small hospital. All of those choices are out there and you can have the job you want! Do you want to go snow skiing and then water skiing? Do you want to be a snowbird and not see the snow at all? Do you like the mountains? Do you like the ocean and the beach? All of these will factor in to your decision.

What state do you want to be in? Me, I prefer the state of confusion most of the time! Well, that, and north in the summer and south in the winter. Is your residence in a "compact" state? That may mean a difference if you only want to go to compact states and not have to get another license, or if you don't mind getting another license you can go wherever you desire. Sometimes where you go is directly related to what locations travel companies have to offer.

Whether you choose a location first or a corporation first will depend on your priorities. What means the most to you? Location, money, benefits, or you're just free as a breeze and don't have a preference?

Location

If location is the most important thing to you, you will need to find the travel company that goes where you want to go. For example, if you want to travel to a hospital in Arizona, you would first find companies that are approved for Arizona contracts. (There are some states and some job registries where only a select number of companies can retain those positions, such as the Arizona Hospital Association.) To find out this information, look on the Internet for the Arizona Hospital Association, go to the website and find the list of companies that provide for the staffing needs in Arizona.

The next step is investigating the hospital and community that you are looking at. Search the Internet for more information. Search area chat rooms and do a search on a messaging program for people in that area. The Chamber of Commerce, City Website, and Craigslist are good places to start.

The best place I have found to gain information about a new location is at http://www.homefair.com/. It is here that you can find information on a cost-of-living comparison, city report, school reports, crime statistics, moving calculator, choosing the right school, and rental furniture. The first place that I start is with the city report. This will give you a good idea of what to expect regarding crime rate, city size, climate, age demographics, and the major employers.

Other useful information that you can find here is the average rent on an apartment and what to expect in salary from the salary calculator.

Another excellent source for information is on http://www.apartment.com/. This is especially useful if you are assisting a company in obtaining your own housing. You can also compare what your company is setting you up in, compared to other housing available in that area. You can also check out www.apartmentratings.com to see if there is anyone happy with the place. Just remember to read the comments and don't necessarily go by the rating. Another thing to remember is that people who are upset are more likely to post a rating than a person who is happy with the place.

This brings up another critical element in choosing a travel company: look at, and ask about, the type of housing each company provides in the area that you are looking at. A lot can be told about a company by their housing. Are you getting a deluxe company with a deluxe apartment, or are you getting an older shack?

The companies who really care about their nurses know that a nurse will only be happy if they feel comfortable and safe in their surroundings. Get to know your surroundings online before accepting any job assignment!

Find out what amenities are available at the apartment or motel. Do they have a pool or spa? What about a workout or weight room? Do they allow pets, and if so, how much does it cost for a pet deposit?

If you travel in a recreational vehicle you definitely want to find out if there are any RV parks close by that accept long-term visitors. I am finding out now that some of the newer parks will only accept you if your vehicle was made in the last ten years.

I work nights and my husband is disabled; therefore, our two main priorities are a hot tub and a place that is quiet during the day.

If you have a child, you might want to find out about what schools are available or what support systems are available for home-schooled children. I also want to know where the local church is and what kind of teen program they have.

Now that we have a company and an area that we would like to go to, the next critical step is to investigate and interview the hospital.

Ask yourself, "What type of hospital am I looking for?" Do you prefer a large hospital, a teaching hospital, or a smaller community hospital? Or...does size really matter?

Are you looking to go to a specific region in the country? Make a list of what you are looking for in a hospital. Even though I came from a small hospital, I really enjoyed my time at the level one trauma center that I worked at in Phoenix, Arizona.

Yes, I definitely was more stressed out, but I was treated as a name and a number. I had a large support system there, which helped out also. Most importantly, I learned that although I prefer a smaller facility, I should not be afraid of a larger facility.

Get out another piece of paper and take notes on your hospital interviews. Keep the notes of all your interviews together in a folder or on a clipboard. If a nurse manager brings up something that you hadn't thought of, add that to your list.

Always know the exact location of the hospital. Know what area of town the hospital is in. Then use that information to check out the crime rate of the hospital area.

I might consider working in a higher crime rate area, but I would not want to live there. Do you have a "high crime" plan of action? My husband would definitely be taking me to work and picking me up. I would much prefer to work in an area of low crime, but the amenities of a bigger hospital and town might be worth the 13-week assignment.

For example, I looked at going to a suburb of Los Angeles. This was after I had spent 13 weeks in Phoenix. No, I wasn't too thrilled about staying and working in a place like that, but the amenities were the reason I would spend 13 weeks there. I would love to take my son to all the sights around Los Angeles, such as Disneyland and Universal Studios.

What system do I use? I call it my "Glendale" system! While working in Northern Phoenix, I lived in the Glendale area. This was about as much crime as I would ever want to get into. So, when I'm looking at a place to go, I always compare it to the Glendale, Arizona crime rate. Maybe you would want to use your hometown as a measure.

Corporation

How big is the unit will you be working on? How many nurses are on duty? What is the nurse-to-patient ratio? Depending on the number of patient and nurses, the charge nurse is required also to take patients. This affects the amount of time they are going to have to assist you if needed. Do they have licensed vocational/practical nurses and/or certified nursing assistants? It makes a big difference if you are a registered nurse and not only have all of your patients to take care of but you also have to take care of all the intravenous medications of another nurse.

Think of unit specific questions also. In the intensive care unit you might want to know the average number of ventilators, how many surgical patients, how many medical patients, or how many cardiac patients are there.

As an emergency room nurse, I would want to know if nursing or respiratory therapy does the electrocardiograms. I want to know if I have an emergency room tech to assist me with dressings and splints. Am I responsible for my lab draws, or do the lab techs come to the emergency room and draw?

In this technology and information age you might want to know what kind of charting is done. Do they chart on paper or on the computer? Do they have care plan problem charting or subjective, objective, assessment, and plan charting?

What about the medication system? Do they have a computerized system like a pyxis? How do I obtain medications “after hours”? The time it takes for you to get that medication may be a little slower if you have to have the house supervisor get the medication, or if the hospital has a 24-hour pharmacist available.

How often do the nurses float and what area would you be expected to float to? Tell them up front if there are any floors that you would not be willing to work on.

Next you will need to know about meals. This is especially true if you work nights. At the small hospitals, the night shift is usually responsible to bring their own supper, but in one place where I worked the night shift received their meals free. Plates of food were left in the refrigerator and we just warmed them up in the microwave at break time. At the larger facility that I worked at, the cafeteria was open for an hour or two.

The next thing that I can think of to ask would be about special uniforms or the color of uniforms. I worked in one nursing home where the nursing assistants wore colors and the medication nurses wore a different color. The charge nurses could wear colored pants, but we had to always wear white tops, because the elderly associated “white” with a professional nurse.

Next, you might want to ask about the town, although you should have done some homework on the town already. What is the population? Do they have a seasonal fluctuation? In central California, I worked in a small city in which they had a great influx during the harvest season. During that time of the year it was also very difficult to find a place to live.

What is the average temperature for the time that you are going to be there? Do they have four actual temperature ranges and seasons, or just hot, hotter, hell, and whew, I can breath again! Is it cold, colder, polar bear, then a few months of defrost? Personally, I'm trying to get this snowbird thing worked out... north in the summer and south in the winter!

What about natural disasters? How many major earthquakes have occurred in the past few years? How many tornadoes or hurricanes? How many times does the creek rise to flood stage? I arrived in Central California the first of November, and during my 13-week contract we had the December 22nd Paso Robles earthquake. I landed in Fort Lauderdale on October 23rd and Wilma landed there October 24th. Although I did miss the Tornado near Nashville, TN by a month, and a tornado in Iowa by 75 miles, I'm probably not the best to give advice on diverting away from natural disasters.

Documentation

You've talked to the hospital, and now you are ready to head off to your new destination. Our recruiter talks to the hospital and the deal is done on their end, but what about the deal on your end?

This is where things get fun. This lovely document, my friend, is called a "contract" or an "agreement." Everything is settled upon verbally, then the contract is drawn up and sent to you. Your first assignment before you get to your destination is to read the fine print of the document that will dictate what your career will be like for the next 13 weeks.

Negotiations with the recruiter can sometimes be a tedious job, but every detail must be dealt with. Your first indication might be to think, "We discussed everything, and it's in there." No! I guarantee you that the first time you do that will be the last time that you do that. I have yet to have a contract that I didn't have to add something to.

Sit down in a quiet place and read your contract, word for word and between the lines. If there is any part that you do not agree with, or have questions about, do *not* sign it until those questions have been answered.

If you have a vacation planned, or if you need certain days off, make sure that you get those dates in writing. It has been my experience that if it is not in writing you may have to just live with the consequences. If it *is* in writing, you are guaranteed those days off.

When you open up your new-hire packet you will find several pages of legal jargon that states that you are going to a hospital or facility to work for a certain amount of time for a certain dollar amount. It says that you are going to act like a professional and that the client-hospital and your travel company are going to treat you like a professional.

The employment relationship is the legal arrangement of the contract. As a staff nurse, you were used to being an "at-will" employee, which means that your continued employment was at the discretion of you and the hospital. As a travel nurse, you will become a "contracted employee." Yes, they can still let you go, but as a contracted employee they are obligated to compensate you for breech of contract.

Another type of relationship between nurse, hospital and agency is called "match-hire," in which the nurse is matched to the hospital, but the nurse is paid directly by the hospital. In this situation, the agency matches you to the hospital. The hospital not only gives you a regular paycheck, but they give the agency a preset dollar amount for your services. Be careful of this situation, because benefits can be very tricky here. The agency can't give you certain benefits because you don't get a regular paycheck from them, and the hospital doesn't give you benefits because you aren't a full-time employee. This situation can cause further confusion between nurse and travel agency when it comes to longevity benefits.

We all should know our professional responsibilities, but because some nurses do not act professionally at all times, those paragraphs have to be added. This part of the contract states that if you cannot show up for your assignment, then you need to call at least two hours before your shift starts. This section also draws the lines of when you, in effect, "voluntarily quit." Although some companies allow for a "lenient" day, most of the time, if you do not show up for the first day, they consider that a voluntary quit. As a protection to the travel company, a clause is added that states that if you act in a careless manner that effects patients or the client hospital, you can and will be turned into the local authorities and state nursing board.

The professional responsibility section is also where you agree to follow the standards set up by the Joint Commission Accreditation of Hospitals Organization (JCAHO), the Occupational Health & Safety Organization (OSHA), and the Nurse Practice Act. This section also includes the fact that you must keep your credentials and licenses that are required for the assignment current. These include documentation that might be needed relating to your nursing qualifications, including ACLS, PALS, TNCC, and State Licenses.

Next you will find your start date, the end date, the facility to which you are assigned, your shift, your on-call time, and your flexibility or floating capabilities. This section might also include whether or not you have guaranteed hours.

If you do not want to float or do not want to be put on call, then make sure that is put into writing. If you do not feel comfortable floating to a certain floor, like O.B. or O.R., then state that in your contract. When reviewing this section of your contract, you also must be mindful that part of a travel nurse's job is to be flexible. This is *your* contract, and you must protect yourself!

Your travel arrangements and lodging arrangements should be next. Listed here will be your permanent home address, and even your temporary address. If applicable, your travel housing stipend amount should also be listed here.

When it comes to your work salary and housing, get everything in writing, and don't ever take anything for granted. If there are days off that you want guaranteed, ask for them in your contract. If floating is a possibility, specify the situations that you will not float; as in the fact that "I don't feel comfortable in ICU or OB," so you put in your contracts that you will not float to ICU or OB. If you want every weekend on or every weekend off or you're willing to work every other weekend, specify that in your contract if that matters to you. Put it in writing whether you wish to work overtime or not.

If there is to be any deduction in pay related to a missed shift, that should also be included. If you are put on call, these deductions should not apply. Make sure that the on-call stipulations are there in the contract.

Included also might be what you are to be paid for a per diem rate. This rate is a fixed rate that is paid to you for food, parking, and other ancillary expenses that you will incur while away from your home state. As of writing this chapter, the maximum allowed by the government is no more than $30 per day. Taxes should be taken out of your hourly rate, but not out of your per diem rate. Companies most often call this a "tax-advantage" program. You will file your taxes in your home state, and will get back most of the money that you paid into another state, but also expect to pay into your own state taxes.

It will also indicate what is included in your housing arrangements. With some companies you will also pay for cable and local phone, but most of them will not pay for those extra utilities. But then again, everything is negotiable in this business!

You cannot get paid unless you turn in your time slips. These time slips are usually faxed to the company that you are contracted with. Some companies have you also mail the original to them, while other companies have you give a copy to the nursing manager. If a company wants certain information on this form, it is also included in this part of the contract.

The last part of the contract might include more legal jargon about benefits, injury on the job, alcohol use, illegal drug use, and the confidentiality clause. All of these important items are included in your contract to protect both you and the company.

In fact, that is the sole purpose of any contract that you have with any company: it is to protect you, the employee, and the company. In this business, verbal agreements mean nothing. Have you ever watched those court shows in the afternoon? *Always,* the judge wants to know if you had it in writing. If it isn't in writing, you just lost. A nice recruiter may be a pleasure to work with, but just remember that they are working for the money they get from handling your contract. Remember, they are no more than nursing salespeople.

And You're Off!

After you have picked out the hospital and travel company you need to prepare for the next assignment. The company will send you another employee packet with many official forms that need to be filled out: forms required by the Occupational Health and Safety Authority, the Internal Revenue Service, and other miscellaneous company forms.

You then need to make sure that your living arrangements and transportation arrangements are all squared away. The travel company usually makes flight arrangements, but you need to also arrange for your personal items to get there. Can you get everything in three suitcases? Some things may have to be shipped by UPS or by a moving company. However, having things moved by a moving company can take away a lot of extra money.

Travel nurses are some of the best shoppers at thrift stores! Take only the bare necessities and then go shopping when you get to your new assignment. If you are going to be living at an apartment complex and do not mind used stuff, watch for what is left beside the dumpsters.

Many treasures have been found there. Not that the items are "bad," but when others move from these complexes you would be amazed at what they leave behind. Just like you, others do not want to drag around stuff, so they leave it behind.

On my first assignment my husband and I found a vacuum cleaner and a futon bed. The lady who put them there came out of her apartment just about that time and asked us if we also wanted her television cabinet. Wow! The cabinet turned out to be a corner television cabinet made out of oak, with room for my son's video games below.

After making the thrift store rounds, *then* go to a discount store to purchase the rest of your necessities. When you leave, you take the important and/or expensive stuff with you as much as possible, sell what you can, take it back to the thrift store for tax credit, or set it back out at the dumpsters for the next traveler.

If you are moving to an extended stay or motel, things are much easier. They usually have pots, pans, and dishes. If not, go back to the thrift store and get a small and a large pot to cook with, and one or two dishes and cups. Do not forget to also get a microwave-safe cooking dish. Before you leave, make sure that your recruiter or housing supervisor tells you exactly what "furnished" will mean for that assignment.

If you are staying at a hotel or extended stay, a necessity is definitely a slow cooker. They will usually have a microwave already in place at the motel or extended stay. With a microwave and slow cooker, you can have hot meals ready when you come home from work.

If you're dragging or driving your home with you, you do not have as many things to "pack up," but you need to load the RV with the necessities before you add your other wants and needs of comfort. Included in your RV, you do not want to forget your coffee maker and slow cooker. It has also been my experience that we ladies cannot forget a bag—or two, or three—with our craft and sewing items. I have even been to a few travel trailers with sewing machines right next to their computer on the "dining" room table. Scrap-booking materials are also necessary for some travel nurses.

Be sure to pack your necessary nursing documents, such as your last tuberculosis test, your hepatitis C immunization records, and any other immunization records that your company required you to list on the forms that you sent in. Even though you probably sent them a copy, always have them available.

Pack at least copies of your certificates, and carry your nursing license with you at all times. Be prepared to produce any other documents that human resources may ask for.

Be sure to call the place where you are supposed to stay and inquire as to whether all the necessary arrangements have been made. There is nothing worse than getting to a place and have them say, "We weren't expecting you." Make sure that the landlord of the apartment complex knows when you are expected to arrive, and arrange a tentative time to meet with him/her. I cannot stress enough the importance of getting all your housing arrangements guaranteed before you get to your assignment. This is where the great recruiter part comes in! Oh, and do not forget that wonderful recruiter's phone number.

Chapter Ten

Preparing For an Adverse Reaction

With each travel assignment, we prepare for the adventure, live the escapade, and then our journey ends, only to perpetuate us on to the next quest. But along our path, we cross over many bridges in the form of emergencies, troubled waters, and even the end of the road. These things are more difficult to face as travelers related to the fact that we are out there on our own and don't have a community or family right there to surround us with comforting thoughts. However, a determined travel nurse doesn't give up; we just pack up and move on down the highway of destiny.

Emergencies Along The Road

In case of a medical emergency, we are taught to dial 911, but who do you call when you are hundreds of miles away from home? Be prepared! Be very prepared!

The first line of defense in case of an emergency is to have an emergency planned for. Not that we really want one to happen, but we don't want one to happen and get caught, as they say, "with our pants down." We certainly don't want to panic.

The first order of business is to have someone to call, like AAA, Good Sam's Emergency Road Service, or OnStarTM. Keep those numbers, usually found on your membership card, in your wallet, above the sun visor, or in your purse.

Important phone numbers to have with you include your nursing recruiter, you bank's number, you car insurance agent's number, and a network of friends along the way.

A network of friends is not only handy to have as a safety feature, but could also be a convenience feature. I have several friends around the country with whom I have worked before that I keep track of, and have even had a few invites for supper and a place to stay.

I wouldn't recommend staying with someone whom you have only met online, but I would definitely stay with someone that I had worked with before.

Of course, meeting other travel nurses along the way for supper is great fun. I have even met other travel nurses after work for breakfast!

If you have not invested in a good nationwide cell phone, now is the time. For years I refused to get one because I had a C.B. and it was free. Although very handy at times, some people just aren't comfortable with a C.B. When I was driving forty miles every day to work, the C.B. was all that I had. The few times that I had problems, I would holler at the trucks to send a policeman or highway patrol.

Have a friend or relative lined up to call every time you stop for gas. I always call my parents along the way so if something does happen to me, they have some idea where to start a search. Of course, you would also want to let that person know what route that you are taking.

Although taking some cash is a good idea, taking too much is not a good idea. Keeping a national ATM card, with access via a pin number, is a must. I carry no more than a hundred dollars cash, and attempt to pay for everything off my debit card, which comes out of my bank account. This also gives me documentation for the tax man.

Before embarking on that next adventure, it is also a necessity to visit your local mechanic to get the oil changed and the fluids checked, along with tire pressure.

In the trunk of your vehicle you should keep extra food, blankets, and water, in the event that you have a roadside emergency.

Make sure that you have a good map. The best maps with nationwide truck stops can be found at the major "chain" truck stops, and some even provide a list of rest areas. Another great resource is the location of tourist information centers as you go into a state. They not only provide you with free maps, but they also have interesting facts about the territory you are about to travel through.

When on a long trip and you haven't ever been that direction, you should always start looking for a gas station when you reach one-half of a tank. By doing this, you don't risk getting too low before finding a place to stop. This is especially essential if you are pulling a travel trailer or traveling in a big motorhome. It is also important to remember that your gas mileage is a lot different when you are pulling a trailer.

When getting out of your vehicle to fill up with gas or go to use the restroom, always be aware of your surroundings. If someone makes you feel uncomfortable, stay in your vehicle and travel to the next rest area if possible.

If you are a female traveling alone, it is not advisable to drive at night, although I do know some women who aren't afraid of traveling alone because their safety is insured by Smith and Wesson.

That brings up the point that if you do have a concealed weapon, be sure that you know the concealed weapon laws in the states you travel through. Other personal safety items to keep in the vehicle consist of a large flashlight, which not only provides light, but can be used as a weapon. They also make a small light that goes on your key chain with an ultraviolet light that will blind someone, giving you time to get out of a dangerous situation.

Another great tip is to carry a device in your glove compartment that will allow you to break the glass or cut your seatbelt in case of a traffic accident.

And last but not least for on the road, always make sure that your spare tire actually has air in it! You wont be too happy if you find this out along the Interstate.

Once you have arrived at your assignment, a phone book with the yellow pages is a must. Look in it to find the nearest urgent care center, the grocery stores, the laundromat, and if you have a pet, an emergency vet. Once you are making good money as a travel nurse, get some of your bills paid off and save up at least enough money to float you for a few months.

In my case, it sure was nice when my dad became sick last year that I had enough saved up to take two months off. In the event of a family emergency, quick airline tickets can be found at www.hotwire.com, priceline.com, and bereavementair.com.

By using these tips and others, you can travel from state to state with peace of mind. By preparing for an emergency, you will know that if something does come up, you won't be the first to hit the panic button, because you will have everything under control

Surviving The Assignment

My patient was screaming down the hallway about how it was time for his pain shot; the nursing supervisor just called and my admit will be here in ten minutes; when I called the surgeon about his patient that is bleeding through his dressing, I got yelled at because I didn't call sooner; and if the patient in room 19 doesn't quit hitting at the staff, then I'm going to have to call his doctor to get an order for restraints; and, of course, there is no one to help me because I'm the traveler, making "all the big bucks." Are travel nurses supposed to think that this is "normal" behavior, or is this nursing abuse?

Pain management is getting to be a bigger and bigger issue. Yes, there are patients who have legitimate pain management needs, but how many patients are we taking care of where this is their second admission this month because they need their morphine fix? This is a bigger issue in the emergency room than I see on the medical-surgical floor. The 1-10 "oucher" scale was supposed to help this, but some patients have figured that out and will rate their pain as a 15.

What are nurses to do about the abuse of the system? We just have to continue to assess our patients in a timely manner and provide them with their medications, as ordered by their physician. There is nothing that we can do about this abuse of the system because we are not that patient and we have been told that we have "no right" to judge how much pain a patient is really in.

Working with physicians that are verbally humiliating, degrading, and have a total lack of respect for us as professional nurses is also a fact in the life of a nurse. In a recent study published by the Association of OR Nurses, over 90% of nurses that were polled were subject to verbal abuse by a physician. Is that true just in the operating room? I don't think so! Trying calling certain physicians in the middle of the night.

What can we do about verbal abuse? What usually happens is that we vent to a few of our co-workers, we keep the patient in mind, and go on and do our job to the best of our abilities. Remember, the patient is why we are there. We must call that physician in the middle of the night to protect our patient, as well as for protection of our license.

Abuse of a nurse by the patient is also a common problem that nurses face during the work day/night. The patient is under the influence of narcotics, illicit drugs, or alcohol and we're supposed to be understanding because they *are* ill. Would they still be ill if they weren't under the influence of all those substances?

We must protect our own health, and when a patient gets violent we need to seek assistance as soon as possible. If we are injured, this needs to be reported to the nursing supervisor as soon as possible, along with getting medical treatment for ourselves.

Do we have the right to press charges against that patient for assault? In some states, a hospital employee definitely has the right to press charges against that patient. There should be no difference if that patient injured us inside the hospital or if he injured us out on the street. If nurses get hurt, who is going to take care of us?

Of course we have to deal with all these things, plus "crises" that occur, and not make any mistakes on these hectic floors. Time management is the key to survival! Come out on the floor, check out your patients and then get a routine going. No, you can't stick by your routine every day. Things happen— patients have surgery, patients have to be admitted—but if you have your routine set up, then it is easier to accomplish these other tasks without getting overwhelmed.

When an overwhelming situation comes along, ask for help. Hostility may be amongst the nursing tribe because you are a travel nurses "making all the big bucks," but you can't do everything by yourself. You need to ask for help. If you can't get anyone to help you, approach the charge nurse and then work your way up the chain of command, all the way to the nursing supervisor. If hostility occurs, contact the director of nursing and your recruiter.

Travel nurses are in hospitals all around the United States and select foreign countries. They are there to help. They are not going to these different places to be abused by other staff and patients. You should be flexible in helping your co-workers, but you don't have to take severe abuse. Keep on working hard, and remember that you only have thirteen weeks there.

Don't be afraid to stand up for yourself. If you become overwhelmed with the pressures to the point that your license is in danger, you must get out of the contract. You were looking for a job when you found that one. Life may have its speed bumps, but just keep on trucking down on the travel-nursing road. The next assignment has to be better!

Looking back at all the tough assignments that I have had, I asked myself, "What are some of the techniques that I use when things are getting tough?" As we all know, travel nursing isn't always fun. We have plenty of good times and adventure, but there are also times when we want to run and hide.

Yes, survival is what it is all about. It's a jungle out there, and a travel nurse must be prepared to tread through the trenches and come out a victor! Come on, there can't be much difference between surviving in a jungle and surviving a terrible nursing assignment. Here are my eight tips for survival in Travel Nursing:

- Shield yourself with a "net" by putting a smile on your face. How can you be sad if you are smiling? Sure, you might be smiling only on the outside, but that is a start. You can shield your patients from knowing that you are having a bad day by wearing a smile!

- Get rid of the leeches! Stay away from the people who are most commonly the causes of the frustration. Sometimes you can't ignore them, but by getting more involved in nursing care and farther away from the nurses' station, the less these leeches will bother you.
- Delve into the trenches. One of the best diversion tactics that I rely on is to spend more time with my patients. Take time out just to visit with them. What can you do for your patients instead of sitting up at the nurses' station, listening to what all is wrong with the unit?
- When the rainfall is heavy, find shelter. You have someone that you can talk to. If nothing else, call your recruiter or get online and find a travel nurse support group. Sometimes things will resolve themselves if you just tell your frustrations to someone who is going to give you a little reassurance.
- In a violent storm or monsoon season, it may be necessary to find a lifeboat. Talk to your recruiter about what is going on. Talk to the unit manager or someone who is over the person that you are having trouble with. If you really feel like your nursing license is in danger, go talk to your recruiter and/or an attorney about getting out of your contract.
- Finding the light in the midst of darkness. Find something that makes you happy and surround yourself with it. Go on a little shopping trip and get something that you have always wanted. Find a place of serenity and immerse yourself in meditation. On bad days I tend to come back to my little "ol'" RV, sit outside, and watch the waterfall that I have in my pond. I would definitely suggest that a travel nurse have some kind of small water feature to travel with her.
- A positive attitude can keep some of the mosquitoes from getting to you. Go into each day with the thought that you are going to make it the best that you can. That may change

twenty minutes into your day, but at least you started out on the right foot.

- Count down the days. Seeing the light at the end of the tunnel is always refreshing. Mark on your calendar the number of weeks left, or even the number of shifts left. Twenty-seven days sounds a lot better than two months!

These tips and tricks may not work for everyone; but for me, they keep me going through tough assignments. Remember that you are there because of your love for nursing, without all the politics. Remember that you do care, and that there will always be the next assignment and another exciting adventure in travel nursing.

Using Laughter To Survive Your Assignment

We've all heard the saying, "Laughter is the best medicine," but just how can it help you through your day as a traveling nurse?

Our first two weeks at a new assignment has to be the toughest. It is at this time that I am trying to adjust to my new surroundings and I want to make an impression that I really do know what I am talking about. In the first weeks I have to prove that I am not into travel nursing just go to from company to company to see how much I can get away with. It is only after establishing that professional relationship that I start mixing in a little humor.

A little humor can go a long ways in making an assignment the best that it can be. Even with my worst assignment, humor is what made my day worth getting up for. Not humor with the other staff members, but humor with my patients. Even though the staff was under a lot of stress and anxiety, my patients were well taken care of and smiling because I was busy taking care of them with a little bit of everyday humor.

On the second day that I have a patient I can usually gain a smile by asking, "Can I listen to see if your heart is beating today?"

This simple attempt at humor will give me a feel about how well the patient is going to accept humor. With some patients that is the start of a wonderful humor relationship, and with others they let me know right quick that they are not in the mood for my little antics.

Some of my most memorable patients haven't been those that are grumpy, but those patients that I have laughed with through their many days at the hospital. Not only does this elevate my patient's mood, but it also has been proven to make a difference in muscle relaxation, neuropeptide release that affects depression, vasodilatation that reduces hypertension, and it also has the most effect on the hardening of attitudes.

Many of the places I have been want me to extend, not only because I'm there to work and do my job, but because of the humor and positive attitude that I bring to the unit.

Someone was fumbling with the foil surrounding a suppository the other day and I just calmly walked over and asked, "You know why they include the directions to take off the foil... because you *know* that someone did *not*." That little chuckle took away some of the stress that she was having opening that silly packaging.

You don't have to be a comedian to be a humorist. Just keep your eyes open to everyday occurrences. Did you ever wonder why they put the instructions on the hemorrhoid cream, "Do not take PO"? Yes! Because someone, somewhere, was eating the hemorrhoid cream and complaining to the company that it wasn't helping their hemorrhoids, and that they couldn't eat anything larger than a jelly bean. And what ever possessed the hospital to contract "Seymour Butts" to design hospital gowns?

Now that you're smiling...take that smile to work and make your co-workers and patients smile right along with you.

Unexpected Contract Termination

What is a nurse to do? What constitutes valid grounds for the nurse to break a contract? What constitutes valid grounds for the travel company to break a contract?

A travel nursing contract is a legally binding contract, and cannot be broken for just any old petty reason. Part of the nursing shortage problem can be from working conditions. Again, document this on your interview information sheet. Unsafe living conditions can include housing that is inhumane or insecure.

As a travel nurse, you need to do your homework on your accommodations before signing the contract. By using http://

www.apartments.com/ or http://www.homefair.com/, apartment and general housing location's crime rates can be checked out. What crime rate is an acceptable crime rate for you? Do *not* hesitate to call security to escort you to your vehicle if you decide to take a job in a higher crime area.

The trend for big problems usually arises with the larger companies that place corporate politics over taking care of their nursing staff. Recruiters can only do so much for their nurses in a larger cooperation. If the problem does not get solved, give them written notice as to why you believe that the contract has been breeched, and that you are terminating your contract due to their breech of contract and their inability to resolve the problem. Health reasons can also be considered as a legitimate reason not to complete a contract.

Serious health problems, such as orthopedic and/or medical problems that require surgical interventions, motor vehicle accidents, or medical problems that will take an extended period of time to recover (i.e. hepatitis) are legitimate reasons to end a contract. If you are not able to complete your contract because of health reasons, the request to terminate the contract early must be in written form, which also need to be accompanied by a physician's statement.

Health reasons for immediate family are also considered a legitimate reason to ask for early termination of a contract.

I don't know of any travel nurse who can say that they have never been homesick at some time in their travel-nursing career. Keep your ears and eyes open for other travel nurses at work.

There are also plenty of online gaming sites, if you enjoy that. Other things that I have found travel nurses love to do are sewing and scrapbooking. If you want to go home for the holidays, then attempt to arrange your contract lengths to give you that time off. Stick to your grounds in following the Nursing Practice Act. Tell the charge nurse what is going on, and tell your recruiter what is going on when problems occur so you have "backup" if the problems get bigger.

Some travel nurses ask for the second floor, related to the noise of the neighbors walking around if they were on the first floor.

This worked fine until one travel nurse noticed that there was a third floor also! Be careful that if this matters to you to ask for the top floor.

Ask your recruiter for a different apartment assignment, and if you absolutely cannot stand it, then you might consider breaking your contract, but this will probably result in major monetary penalties.

You have an agreement with the travel company that is a legal and binding contract. Problems can usually be ironed out along the way by talking to the nurse manager or your recruiter.

Chapter Eleven

Keeping Track Of Important Tax Information

Once a year, we have the task of filing our taxes and paying to Uncle Sam what we owe in support of our government. As a traveling nurse, special rules apply to what you can and what you cannot take out as a travel expense.

Travel expenses are defined as "the ordinary and necessary expenses of traveling away from your home for business." Generally, employees can deduct their expenses using the 2106 form provided by the Internal Revenue Service, which is titled "Employee Business Expenses." However, you cannot deduct expenses that are lavish or extravagant or that are for personal purposes.

To take out these expenses, you must sign a contract to work away from home for a period substantially longer than an ordinary day's work, and need to get sleep or rest to meet the demands of your work while away. Contrary to myth, there is no "50 mile" rule.

You are traveling away from home if:

1. Your duties require you to be away from the general area of your tax home substantially longer than an ordinary day's work, and
2. You need to sleep or rest to meet the demands of your work while away from home.

This rest requirement is not satisfied by merely napping in your car. You do not have to be away from your tax home for a whole day, or from dusk to dawn, as long as your relief from duty is long enough to get the necessary sleep or rest.

For example, if you are working 70 miles from home and drive back home for the night before returning to work the next day, you are considered to be commuting to work, not traveling to work, because you returned home for rest. In this case, all income and subsides will be taxable income.

If you are working 100 miles from home and drive back home on your days off, then the expenses you incur are tax deductible because you have to rent a place to sleep on the days that you work to receive adequate rest. If you rent a place for 7 days a week at the work site, all the lodging expenses are deductible, even for the days that you returned home.

The same applies for a travel assignment in that if you travel and stay at a place for thirteen weeks, then your travel to the assignment, expenses during the assignment related to work, and travel back home or to your next assignment are all tax deductible. During the assignment, you can deduct the expenses for trips home, but only up to the amount that you would have deducted had you stayed at the work site.

There are no rules about how often you have to return to you home, but it is a good idea to return home often. Either you are traveling for a living or you are away from home. If you are away from home, you will not abandon your home. To determine whether you are traveling away from home, you must first determine the location of your tax home.

Tax Home

Your tax home is generally the place where your permanent home is, if you have a permanent house. Keep in mind also that if you do not have a regular place of doing business or a conventional home, then you are considered a "transient" and your tax home is wherever you work. This has a drawback in the fact that you cannot declare travel costs as a deduction because you are never considered to be traveling away from home.

According the IRS publication 463, generally, your tax home is your regular place of business or post of duty, regardless of where you maintain your family home. It includes the entire city or general area in which your business or work is located. If you do not have a regular or a main place of business because of the nature of your work, your tax home may be the place where you regularly live.

If you do not have a regular place of business or post of duty and there is no place where you regularly live, you are considered an "itinerant" or a "transient" and your tax home is wherever you work. As an itinerant, you cannot claim a travel expense deduction because you are never considered to be traveling away from home.

If you have more than one place of work, consider the following when determining which one is your main place of business or work:

- The total time you ordinarily spend in each place.
- The level of your business activity in each place.
- Whether your income from each place is significant or insignificant.

A tax home must consist of a habitable dwelling. This means that a storage shed or piece of land cannot be considered a tax home. The piece of land must have a structure on it in which you can sleep, cook, and have a restroom. In other words, you must have a self-contained domestic establishment. The same thing is true with a storage shed; unless you build a special shed with living quarters, it cannot be counted as a home. In no way can a mailbox be considered a tax home. You cannot live in a mailbox.

In addition to having a place to live, you must have direct ties to the community that you call your tax home. A strong financial and legal connection, such as a checking account, driver's license, car registration, and mail service is a must for a tax home.

You can use your parents' address, but you must pay them to rent a room while you are away on assignment. To accomplish this, you need to find out what the market value is for the area in which your parents live. What is a studio type of apartment going for or a room for rent? After you find out what the room rate is, I would suggest that you have a contract signed between you and your parents (or other relative), stating how much you are paying to cover the rental and utility charges. Then you must actually pay your parents for the room, and they must claim the rental income on their income taxes.

Be careful to protect your tax home, for all that it is worth. While on assignment, don't change your driver's license, car registration, or other license tags to your temporary address. All bank accounts, credit cards, monthly bills, and other debts that you pay every month should have your permanent home address on them instead of your temporary address. To make bill paying easier while on the road, it is a great idea to pay your bills using the Internet, or have automatic withdrawals for things like your vehicle and house payment.

If at all possible, have your company send your W-2 to your permanent address and list that address on the form. This is not always possible with most payroll arrangements.

Transportation, Meals, and Incidentals

You can also deduct the expense of meals if it is necessary for you to stop for substantial sleep, or that the meal is business-related. These meals cannot be lavish or extravagant. A standard meal allowance is provided to you, based on where your business away from your home is conducted.

According to IRS Publication 463, "You can use the actual cost of your meals to figure the amount of your expense before reimbursement and application of the 50% deduction limit. If you use this method, you must keep records of your actual cost. Generally, you can use the "standard meal allowance" method as an alternative to the actual cost method. It allows you to use a set amount for your daily meals and incidental expenses (M&IE), instead of keeping records of your actual costs. The set amount varies, depending on where and when you travel. In this publication, "standard meal allowance" refers to the federal rate for M&IE, discussed later under "Amount of standard meal allowance." If you use the standard meal allowance, you still must keep records to prove the time, place, and business purpose of your travel.

The standard meal allowance in the year of 2006 was at least $39 per day in the United States. Some metropolitan areas will have more elevated standards; such as Los Angeles, California, where you are allowed $64 per day for food. The standard meal allowance for your locality can be found at http://www.gsa.gov/perdiem. To find a further breakdown of how much you are allowed for each meal, visit: www.gsa.gov/mie/. For example, for $39/day you are allowed $7 for breakfast, $11 for lunch, $18 for supper, and $3 for incidentals. The website also breaks it down for those cities which are allowed $44, $49, $54, $59, and $64.

Transportation expenses deductions can be taken on expenses related to getting from your home to a temporary workplace when you have one or more regular places of work. If you have one or more regular work locations away from you home and you commute to a temporary work location in the same profession, you can deduct the expenses of the daily round-trip transportation between your home and the temporary location, regardless of distance.

Remember also that a temporary work assignment is considered an assignment that is expected to last less than one year; the employment is temporary unless there are facts that would indicate otherwise. As a travel nurse, all assignments are considered temporary unless you stay in the same metropolitan area for more than 12 months. This period of time is measured by continuous employment or a series of assignments with short breaks. Repetitive assignments in the same area can shift your tax home. .

You may also take out a mileage expense. The standard mileage rate for 2006 is 48.5 cents a mile. This rate is adjusted every one or two years to concur with the greater cost-of-living factor. The standard mileage rate not only considers the amount that you spend on gas, but the upkeep and "wear and tear" on your vehicle. To find the current rate, go to: www.gsa.gov/mileage/.

A word of caution: there is no optional standard lodging amount similar to the standard meal allowance. Your allowable lodging expense deduction is your actual cost. Incidental expenses, according to the IRS Publication 463 are

1. Fees and tips given to porters, baggage carriers, bellhops, hotel maids, stewards or stewardesses and others on ships, and hotel servants in foreign countries;
2. Transportation between places of lodging or business and places where meals are taken, if suitable meals can be obtained at the temporary duty site; and
3. Mailing costs associated with filing travel vouchers and payment of employer-sponsored charge card billings.

Incidental expenses do not include expenses for laundry, cleaning and pressing of clothing, lodging taxes, or the costs of telegrams or telephone calls.

Other important things to remember about your travel include new rules that apply to the days of travel that you depart and return. (For both the day you depart and the day you return from a business trip you must prorate the standard meal allowance (figure a reduced amount for each day). You can do so by one of of these two methods.

- You can claim ¾ of the standard meal allowance.
- You can prorate, using any method that you consistently apply and that is in accordance with reasonable business practice.

As far as mixing business with pleasure, the IRS has this to say: "You can deduct all of your travel expenses if your trip was entirely business-related. If your trip was primarily for business and while at your business destination you extended your stay for a vacation, made a personal side trip, or had other personal activities, you can deduct your business-related travel expenses. These expenses include the travel costs of getting to and from your business destination and any business-related expenses at your business destination.

If your trip was primarily for personal reasons, such as a vacation, the entire cost of the trip is a non-deductible personal expense. However, you can deduct any expenses you have while at your destination that is directly related to your business.

A trip to a resort or on a cruise ship may be a vacation, even if the promoter advertises that it is primarily for business. The scheduling of incidental business activities during a trip, such as viewing videotapes or attending lectures dealing with general subjects, will not change what is really a vacation into a business trip.

Record Keeping

As a travel nurse, you will be responsible for keeping track of all of the expenditures related to your travel. Lack of organization throughout the year in this business is considered a medical emergency! You *must* keep track of things. You *must* plan at least one day every week or two weeks to write everything down in a journal or enter it into a computer program such as QuickenTM or MoneyTM. You can also do things the "old fashioned" way and log everything into a journal.

The program I use allows me to keep track of everything, taxable and non-taxable. It helps me keep track of all the money I have going in and coming out. I even have a table set up on a spreadsheet program that helps me keep track of my mileage, since I am traveling every two weeks to and from my assignment and my residence. In fact, the new version of Quicken 2004, report that they are also able to keep track of your mileage!

Keeping track of receipts for everything is also very important. The best way to do that is to purchase one of those plastic hanging file folder storage systems. In fact, I have four of those that I travel with—one with my online business papers, one with my travel nursing papers, one with personal business papers, and one for all my craft and sewing patterns. Organization is the key to successful travel nursing!

If you deduct travel, entertainment, gift, or transportation expenses, you must be able to prove (substantiate) certain elements of those expenses. If you keep timely and accurate records, you will have support to show the IRS if your tax return is ever examined. You will also have proof of expenses that your employer may require if you are reimbursed under an accountable plan.

You should keep adequate records to prove your expenses or have sufficient evidence that will support your own statements. You must generally prepare a written record for it to be considered adequate. This is because written evidence is more reliable than oral evidence alone. However, if you prepare a record in a computer memory device with the aid of a logging program, it is considered an adequate record.

You should keep the proof you need in an account book, diary, statement of expense, or similar record. You should also keep documentary evidence that, together with your record, will support each element of an expense.

Documentary evidence ordinarily will be considered adequate if it shows the amount, date, place, and essential character of the expense.

For example, a hotel receipt is enough to support expenses for business travel if it has all of the following information:

- The name and location of the hotel.
- The dates you stayed there.
- Separate amounts for charges such as lodging, meals, and telephone calls.

A restaurant receipt is enough to prove an expense for a business meal if it has all of the following information:

- The name and location of the restaurant.
- The number of people served.
- The date and amount of the expense.

If a charge is made for items other than food and beverages, the receipt must show that this is the case.

You should record the elements of an expense or of a business use at or near the time of the expense or use and support it with sufficient documentary evidence. A timely kept record has more value than a statement prepared later, when generally there is a lack of accurate recall.

You do not need to write down the elements of every expense on the day of the expense. If you maintain a log on a weekly basis that accounts for use during the week, the log is considered a timely-kept record. You must generally provide a written statement of the business purpose of an expense. However, the degree of proof varies, according to the circumstances in each case. If the business purpose of an expense is clear from the surrounding circumstances, then you do not need to give a written explanation.

If you do not have complete records to prove an element of an expense, then you must prove the element with

- Your own written or oral statement containing specific information about the element, and
- Other supporting evidence that is sufficient to establish the element.

If the element is the description of a gift, or the cost, time, place, or date of an expense, the supporting evidence must be either direct evidence or documentary evidence. Direct evidence can be written statements or the oral testimony of your guests or other witnesses, setting forth detailed information about the element. Documentary evidence can be receipts, paid bills, or similar evidence.

If the element is either the business relationship of your guests or the business purpose of the amount spent, the supporting evidence can be circumstantial, rather than direct. For example, the nature of your work, such as making deliveries, provides circumstantial evidence of the use of your car for business purposes. Invoices of deliveries establish when you used the car for business.

Employees who give their records and documentation to their employers and are reimbursed for their expenses generally do not have to keep copies of this information. However, you may have to prove your expenses if any of the following conditions apply:

- You claim deductions for expenses that are more than reimbursements.
- Your expenses are reimbursed under a non-accountable plan.
- Your employer does not use adequate accounting procedures to verify expense accounts.

Hopefully, this chapter will help provide answers to some of your questions concerning travel taxes. I would also strongly suggest that you go to the IRS' website and download the latest copy of Publication 463. This is your "Travel Tax Bible" and could save you thousands of dollars every year!

On the next page you will find a form that will assist you in keeping track of all of your important tax information. For each assignment, fill out this form.

Assignment Information:

Assignment City: ______________________________
Assignment Dates: ____/____/____ to ____/____/____
Travel Company: ______________________________
Mileage to assignment: __________________________
Commuting mileage: ____________________________
Mileage home from assignment: __________________
Airfare: _____________________________________
Truck or Trailer Moving Rental: _________________
Car Rental: ___________________________________
Other Miscellaneous Expenses: __________________

Miscellaneous Business Fees:
Parking Fees: _________________________________
Mass Transit Fees: _____________________________
Tolls: ____
Laundry: _____________________________________
Continuing Education Fees: ____________________
State Licensing Fees Not Reimbursed: ____________
Association Dues: ______________________________
Professional Publications & Journals: ____________
"Land Line" Charges: ___________________________
Cell Phone Charges: ____________________________
Malpractice insurance: _________________________
Cable Service Fees: _____________________________

~*~

Travel Tax Updates from 2007 & 2008

The Tax Relief and Health Care Act has some new tax law changes that went into effect in 2007 and 2008, including:

1) Most of the expiring deductions have been renewed—the tuition and fees, educator, state and local sales tax deductions have all been renewed and are always subject to change.
2) Beginning Jan 1 2007, mortgage insurance premiums became deductible for any new loans. This adds to the tax deductions already allowed for mortgage interest and real estate taxes. These loans must be taken out in 2007 or later.
3) A tax-free rollover of funds from IRAs to Health Savings Accounts is allowed once during a person's lifetime. The contribution is limited to the maximum amount that you could contribute during the year and reduced by any contributions that you make for the year that you initiate the rollover. This is a round about method of funding an HSA for the first year.
4) Any unused amounts in Flexible Spending Accounts (FSAs) or Health Reimbursement Arrangements (HRAs) can be rolled into an HSA.
5) Know a tax cheat? New laws increase the rewards for reporting tax fraud.
6) Starting with 2007, charitable donations *must* have a receipt. The IRS will no longer accept logs or other forms of documentation, even for donations to the Salvation Army kettles. When dropping off clothes, etc., list the items and get some form of a receipt from the attendant.
7) For those of you working as contractors, incorporation will be the norm in the future. IRS regulations and liability issues are forcing many agencies to require a healthcare professional working as an independent contractor to incorporate, hence employ themselves.
8) For those starting HSA accounts with high deductible health plans, you can fund these accounts with a one time, penalty free rollover from your IRA to an HAS Duplicate of #3.

9) Unless Congress cleans up the AMT (Alternative Minimum Tax) issues, many more middle income taxpayers will be hit by this 2nd tax rate. More and more travelers are affected by this each year.
10) Corporate taxpayers should remember that a reasonable salary must be paid first *before* paying any profits as dividends. This is a hot topic for the IRS.
11) Mutual Fund Distributions: A recent court case determined that the IRS was wrong in imposing capital gains taxes on the full amount of stock proceeds from life insurance companies to their policy holders. If you received a stock distribution from an insurance company and paid taxes on the distribution, you may be due for a refund.
12) First Time Home Buyer Credit: A new "credit" for first-time home buyers has been passed, but beware; you have to pay it back over 15 years. If you have not owned a home in the last 3 years and purchase a dwelling between April 9, 2008 and June 30, 2009, you can get a 10% tax credit for the purchase price. The credit is limited to $7500 and may be claimed in the following year on the tax return. There are other stipulations, but again, payback is required so it is not as great a credit.
13) Property Tax Credit: New legislation allows single non-itemizers to deduct up to $500 in real property taxes and married filing jointly non-itemizers up to $1000 in real property taxes. The deduction is only available for 2008.
14) (For Canadian Travelers) New tax laws in Canada have created a Tax Free Savings Account (TFSA) similar to the ROTH IRAs in the US, only it is not a retirement account, but a general savings account for items like home purchases, or even a family vacation. Taxpayers and their spouses can contribute 5K a year and any contribution room can be carried to the next year. The contributions are not deductible, but the earnings grow tax free. Additionally, any withdrawals can be restored without

affecting contribution limits. These accounts can be opened at any financial institution.

15) (For Canadian Travelers) Quebec now recognizes US Social Security Taxes as a tax credit. If you were a Quebec resident and worked in the US in 2004 or later, you may be able to claim a refund on for Social Security taxes paid to the US on your QC return.
16) (For Canadian Travelers) RRSPs and IRAs treated equally. Remember that you can now take a deduction on your US or Canadian return (your resident nation) for retirement contributions in the other nation. The new treaty protocols issued late in 2007 simplified this issue.

Big thanks to Joseph Smith, RRT, EA of www.traveltax.com for his expert advice and professional editing of this chapter. His experience as an IRS Enrolled Agent and respiratory therapist experience makes him a valuable asset for travel nursing tax information. Thank you for keeping us updated through the year!

~*~

For more information, check with the Internal Revenue Service's website at: www.irs.gov Parts of this chapter were directly taken from this public website which states "Content on this web site that was created or maintained by Federal employees in the course of their duties is not subject to copyright and may be freely copied."

Chapter Twelve
Going at It All Alone

Many nurses now have put on the hat of nurse entrepreneur. Getting contracts by yourself and doing your own independent contracting is a little tougher than just having an agency helping you with taxes, government dues, insurance, and getting assignments, but there are definite advantages, with more money coming into your pocket and having control over your destination.

One of the basic differences of being an independent contractor instead of an employee is that you will be receiving the IRS Form 1099 instead of a W2 form. This IRS Form 1099 shows the amount that was paid for services rendered. This form will have on it the account number (or unique number), the payer assigned to distinguish your account, the amount subject to self-employment taxes, other income, backup withholdings, and any state of local income tax withheld from the payments.

Another difference is that you will be responsible for obtaining your own contracts. Most commonly, this is done in two ways: First, by calling the hospital and seeing the availability of contracts, which they usually use for contracts, and if they would consider an independent contract, or you can contact a company that specializes in independent contracts. These companies will charge you a few dollars per hour for helping you in obtaining a "subcontract" through them. Some of the companies who do subcontracting include: Attentive Healthcare (www.attentivehealthcare.net), CMSI (www.travelrn.com), Comforce (www.comforcetravelrn.com), Hospital Support (www.hospitalsupport.com), Independent Nurse Consultants (www.independentnurse.com).

I know, you're anxious to get down the road by yourself, but there are just a few more basics that you have to understand, such as the type of business you are going to have, formulating a business plan, creating a marketing plan, must have's for the office, and what to put into the contract. You just never know, after starting your own independent contractor business, you may want to expand and let other nurses share in your happiness and wealth.

What Type of Business?

First, you need to decide what type of business you will start. There are several types, including a sole proprietor (the most common), a C-Corporation, an S-Corporation, or a limited liability corporation (LLC).

A Sole proprietorship is a corporation that officially has no separate existence from its owner. Hence, the limitations of liability enjoyed by a corporation do not apply. All debts of the business are debts of the owner. It is a "sole" proprietor in the sense that the owner has no partners. A sole proprietorship essentially means that a person does business in their own name and there is only one owner. A sole proprietorship is not a corporation; it does not pay corporate taxes, but rather the person who organized the business pays personal income taxes on the profits made, making accounting much simpler. A sole proprietorship need not worry about double taxation like a corporation would have to.

A business structured as a sole proprietorship will likely have a hard time creating capital, since shares of the business cannot be sold, and there is a smaller sense of legitimacy relative to a business that is organized as a corporation or limited liability company. Hiring employees may also be difficult. This form of business will have unlimited liability; therefore, if the business is sued, it is the proprietor's problem.

Another disadvantage of a sole proprietorship is that as a business becomes successful, the risks accompanying the business tend to grow. To minimize those risks, a sole proprietor has the option of forming a limited liability company. Most sole proprietors will register a trade name or "Doing Business As" with (with whom?). This allows the proprietor to do business with a name other than their legal name, and it also allows them to open a business account with banking institutions.

A C-corporation is a form of corporation that meets the IRS requirements to be taxed under Subchapter C-of the Internal Revenue Code. Most major companies are incorporated under a C-corporation. After the corporation is created, it becomes its own entity and has an indefinite lifespan, as long as the yearly filing fee is paid. This is what you would want to file if you were starting a staffing agency that would have several employees.

The main difference between S and C lie in the fact that a C-corporation is taxed a Federal Corporate Income tax, whereas an S-corporation is not. It may also have an unlimited amount of shareholders, as well as foreign shareholders, unlike S-corporations.

In order to accomplish the task of becoming a C-Corp, you will need to choose an available business name that complies with your state's corporation rules, appoint the initial directors of your corporation, file formal paperwork, usually called "articles of incorporation," and pay a filing fee that ranges from $100 to $800, depending on the state in which you incorporate, create corporate "bylaws," which lay out the operating rules for your corporation, hold the first meeting of the board of directors, issue stock certificates to the initial shareholders of the corporation, and obtain licenses and permits that may be required for your business.

An S-Corporation is taxed as a joint venture, while at the same time it enjoys the benefit of incorporation. This means that while the S-Corporation itself pays no federal income tax, the shareholders of the S-Corporation pay federal income tax on their proportionate share of the S-Corporation's income. In other words, any profits earned by the corporation will not be taxed at the corporate level, but instead will be taxed only at the level of the individual shareholders.

Unlike C-Corp dividends, which are taxed at the federal rate of 15.00%, S-Corp Dividends are taxed at the shareholder's marginal tax rate. However, the C-Corp Dividend is subject to "double-taxation." The income is first taxed at the corporate level before it is distributed as a dividend. The dividend is then taxed at the personal capital gains rate when issued to the shareholder.

S-Corp Distributions are only taxed once at the marginal rate of each shareholder who received a distribution. Additionally, the S-Corp shareholder will pay taxes on the S-Corp earnings, whether or not a distribution is made. Having S corporation status can prove a huge benefit for a corporation. The corporation can pass income directly to shareholders and avoid the double taxation that is inherent with the dividends of public companies, while still enjoying the advantages of the corporate structure.

In order to qualify, a corporation must be a small business corporation. Requirements that must be met include the fact that it must be a domestic corporation, must have no more than 100 shareholders, and all of the shareholders must be citizens of the United States. The corporation also must have only one class of stock, and profits and losses must be allocated to shareholders proportionately to each one's interest in the business.

If a corporation meets the foregoing requirements, its shareholders may file Form 2553 with the IRS. The Form 2553 must be signed by all of the corporation's shareholders. If a corporation that has elected to be treated as an S Corporation ceases to meet the requirements, the corporation will lose its S Corporation status.

A Limited Liability Corporation is a legal form of business offering limited liability to its owners. It is similar to a corporation, and is often a more flexible form of ownership, especially suitable for smaller companies with restricted numbers of owners.

An LLC allocates for the flexibility of a sole proprietorship or partnership arrangement within the structure of limited liability, such as that approved for corporations. A benefit of an LLC over a limited partnership is that the rules and regulations required for forming and registering LLCs are much easier than the requirements most states place on developing and managing corporations; most LLCs will; however, decide to implement an Operating Agreement or Limited Liability Company Agreement to provide for the authority of the Company, and such Arrangement is normally more multifaceted than a corporation's statutes.

One motive that an industry might prefer to be planned out as an LLC is to circumvent dual assessment of taxes. A conventional corporation is taxed on its income, and then when the profits are dispersed to the owners of the corporation or shareholders, those dividends are also taxed. With an LLC, income of the LLC is not taxed, but each owner of the LLC is taxed, based on its pro rata allocable portion of the LLC's taxable income, apart from whether any distributions to the associates are made. This single level of taxation can lead to significant savings over the corporate form.

Another underlying principle that a company might choose to be arranged as an LLC is to take advantage of the tax classification flexibility that LLCs allow. A new business facing losses might opt to function as a sole proprietorship or partnership in order to bypass those losses to the owners. A slightly more established business might operate as an S corporation to save on self-employment taxes. A large, mature business with many owners might operate as a C corporation.

Formulating A Business Plan

Your business plan will need to include an executive summary, general company description, products and services, an operation plan, management and organization, a personal financial statement, startup expenses and capitalization, a financial plan, and refining the plan.

The executive summary actually needs to be written last. It should include everything that you would put into a five-minute interview, including the fundamentals of the proposed business, what your services will be, who your customers will be, who the owners are, and what you think the future holds for your business. This summary needs to be KISSed...Keep It So Simple!

The general company description needs to include the fact that you are a registered nurse, providing services to hospitals, and how you will provide those services. You will need a mission statement, usually 40 words or less, which explains your reason for starting this company and what philosophies have guided you to make the decision to strike out on your own.

Next, you will need to state your goals and objectives. What goal do you have for your company? Do you want to be in the Fortune 500, or do you just want to provide great service to others, giving them quality service instead of quantity? This will depend on whether or not you decide to remain a sole proprietor or if you incorporate as a C, S, or Limited Liability Corporation.

To whom are you going to market your products? Hospitals, nursing homes, physicians' offices, surgical centers? What is the future of your company? What changes do you see in the future? How will you deal with those changes?

Also, in the goals and objectives you will need to describe why you think that your company is the best company for the job? Customer service? Experience? Skills?

This is where you will also want to state what type of corporation you have filed as and why you decided to file as that type of corporation.

Next, you will describe in-depth your products or services with technical specifications: what set of skills are available, what can you do for the hospital or medical facility? Which of these features will give you the competitive edge and exclusivity? What is the bill rate for your services? Why is your bill rate a good bargain? Hospitals are looking for the best rates and the best quality together. Can you supply that demand? (This will be discussed further in the marketing plan section).

Next is the operation plan. This will explain the day-to-day operation of the business, its home-base location, people, and processes. Some of the things you will want to include in this section are the services you will provide, quality control aspects, and customer service. Where will your home base be located? Unless you are planning on hiring a lot of nurses in a staffing company type of setting, this will be the physical location of your permanent residence. What type of licensing and insurance will you be carrying on yourself and/or personnel?

If you plan on hiring other nurses, you will need to list how many nurses you will start out with, the units of the hospital that you would like to provide services for, how to pay for their services, training methods, and requirements for nurses, job description, and any need for subcontracted workers.

How will you manage your accounts receivable? You will have to formulate a plan to bill the hospital, as well as how to receive the payments. Independent contractors typically bill the hospital weekly, but payment is usually made only once a month.

Next, you should state your management members and any consults regularly used. Consults that you are smart to have available include an attorney, accountant, insurance agent, banker, nursing profession consultants, small business consultants, and mentors as you feel are needed to help you run a successful business.

After that, you should explain what you believe your startup expenses are, your financial ability to assist with those expenses, and any other capital funds you have acquired or have a plan to acquire. Do your research on exactly how much it is going to cost you to start up a home office. Do you have a computer, fax machine, copy machine, and phone? A fairly inexpensive printer can do faxing, copying, and scanning. Other services can be provided through an office supply store. Once you estimate your start up expenses, it's a general rule to plan on a twenty percent financial pad for unexpected incidentals. How much do you plan to make in a year? How much do you plan to make in five years? What are your long-term financial goals? Do you plan on starting as a sole proprietor and then further incorporate into a Limited Liability Corporation or C-Corp?

Refine your plan to include the key competitive factors in the industry, capacity limits, purchasing and inventory management of supplies, new services under development. How will you manage rapidly changing prices or costs, and how will you remain on the cutting edge with your services?

The preceding questions can be answered by taking your time and doing an in-depth look into what you really want to accomplish with your services as an independent contractor. Having this documentation will give your company more validity.

Creating a Marketing Plan

The purpose of a marketing plan is to put onto paper why you think your product is better than other products, why hospitals should hire you, why hospitals should hire your staff, and the future plans of your company. This plan will assist you in knowing where you have been and where you are going. It will keep your eyes focused on the job at hand—building your travel nursing company into a prosperous and successful business.

We are going to build this nursing company just like we take care of our patients—through assessment, planning, implementation, and evaluation. To accomplish this, first we need to assess what types of services we are going to provide, to whom we are providing those services, who are our competitors, and how the market fluctuates.

What types of services are you going to provide? This will be directly linked to what your nursing specialty is. Are you going to employ others? If you have multiple specialties, then the greatest demand will determine what services you will have the most success in providing to your clients. You will need to do some research into what hospitals you are going to target at first and determine what their needs are.

You need to research what other nursing contractors are out there and what their targeted hospitals are. What do they provide to the hospital that you could provide better? You must declare what the market is lacking in order to determine how you can fill that place.

By doing some research, you can also find out what your competitors are paying. If you explain that you are a nurse wanting to do a travel assignment and wanting to know what types of jobs they have and what the pay rates are, then you can figure a ballpark range of what the bill rate is by taking what they are paying the travel nurses and adding 20% (take the pay rate and multiple it by 1.2). You can also go to salary.com and see what the nursing salary is for that position. To get an idea of a bill rate from this, if you understand that travel nurses make approximately 20% more an hour than staff nurses and the company will also get 20%. By taking the pay rate and multiplying it by 1.4 you can figure out an approximate bill rate.

Your plan will include aligning the price with the apparent value with the customer. If your price seems a little high, drop it a few dollars per hour. If you are unable to get contracts after discussing the bill rate with human resources, you may have to look at changing the price. Keep in mind also that if you provide outstanding service to a customer, you can raise your price a little on the next contract.

Snoop around and see what other competitors are out there. Are there several independent nursing companies available? Are they all providing service to one hospital, or do they cater to a group of hospitals? What are their strengths? What are their weaknesses? How can you capitalize on those weaknesses? Maybe the hospital needs a more flexible nurse... maybe they need someone to work night or weekends... Find out the need and what needs are not being provided for by other nurses and you will get your foot in the door.

You need to plan how you are going to get the word out to these hospitals. There are several ways to get the information into hospitals by using phone calls followed up with brochures and postcards telling hospitals of your new services. Carry business cards with you at all times. You never know when you are talking with people out in the community and you can tell about some hospital, clinic, or nursing home that is "terribly short-staffed, I just don't know how they make it." Your eyes and ears should be open at all times for marketing possibilities.

What are the goals of your marketing efforts, and in what time frame do you want to accomplish them? Some nurses just want a contract for the next month, some want a contract for the next week, and some want a contract for the next year. Do you plan on helping other nurses find contracts? You might have a goal of 10 nurses this year to work in an attempt to make a good living with your company and propel it to the next level.

You also need a plan to launch your business. Follow your business plan and get your business license, get a bank account set up, and have your marketing plan ready to go. A great way to announce the beginning of your company is to place an ad in the newspaper, or better yet, send out press releases in an effort to have the media do a human interest story about why you are starting your own nursing company. If you have a self-contract, you might contact the local newspaper and offer a free article to the newspaper, with your contact and company information as a tag line.

Next, you can implement your plan in attempt to sway the client from a stage of knowledge to one of contemplation. The client needs to have confidence that you will supply their facility with the best of service.

To do this, you will need a set plan, telling when you can start, how much the bill rate will be, how you plan on doing quality control on yourself, and reinforce the fact that the independent contractors services are the best for that client. Work with the client and negotiate for the best possible deal for both you and the client.

Choose where you want to be, and beat down the doors of every hospital in that area by sending out your profile. The profile will include your resumé and a skills checklist, then start your circle to the outskirts of town. Persistence will pay off, and you will find you a job where you want if you put enough time and effort into it.

What To Put Into The Contract

Independent contracts are very similar to those of an agency nurse, but there are some differences that you need to be aware of concerning certain responsibilities: billing, insurance, and other documentation. The following is a brief description of what needs to be included.

The contractor responsibilities: The fact that a contractor (the independent contractor) is to provide nursing services in a certain area of the hospital, according to standards set forth by the Joint Commission on Accreditation for Health Care Organization (JCAHO) and the Nursing Practice Act of the State of Idaho (my home state, you can insert yours).

The contractor certifies and will provide legal documentation of skills acquired in the past 16 years as a licensed nurse, health certificates, personal identification, company identification, and proof of liability insurance with minimum amounts of $1,000,000 per occurrence and $5,000,000 yearly.

This contract will be entered into as n independent contract with the agent not entitled to any benefits accorded to hospital employees, including workman's compensation, disability, vacation, and sick pay.

The client is responsible for providing a safe work environment, including a job description and basic orientation to medication administration, documentation, order transcription, patient safety, and on-the-job employee safety.

You may also put in there the cancellation policy for low census days, areas that you will and will not work based on competency, any guaranteed hours, and nurse-to-patient ratios that are acceptable. Also, add in a phrase about the need to notify you two hours in advance of cancellation and you will notify them two hours in advance of unable to meet the obligation related to an illness.

Next are the financial items, including bill rates, overtime rates, weekend rates, and holiday rates. It is definitely best to keep this simple by charging a basic bill rate, overtime and 1.5 times the base pay, and holiday rates at 1.5 times the base pay. Other things that you can add, if you really feel the need to, are charge nurse pay, weekend pay, and shift differential. Just keep in mind, the more straight-forward and uncomplicated the contract appears, the better it is, but don't cheat yourself either.

You should also add in a statement about when accounts are receivable. Some hospitals only pay out once a month, but by offering a 2-5% discount, some will go with a bi-weekly pay rate. Also, add a section on how much interest will be charged if the amount is not received in a timely manner. This may be anywhere from 2-5% of the total invoice for every day that is late. Also include a statement that if things go to court, lawyer fees will be asked for. You must also state when the work week is—from Sunday to Saturday or from Monday to Sunday. You may have to be negotiable with this and go with the same schedule as the hospital has for their other employees.

Last is the termination clause. This should list how long the contract is to last, and under what circumstance the contract can be terminated. The industry standard is that contracts can be cancelled with or without cause by providing thirty days written notice.

After the basic contract is written, don't be surprised if it goes through a few changes and negotiations with the hospital. It will take you an average of two weeks from the start of the negotiation process to being on the job.

Taxes and Payroll

There are several payroll taxes/costs for the independent contractor to consider ways of minimizing. I'm not including income tax in this definition. Payroll taxes usually refer to FICA, workman's comp, and unemployment insurance.

The biggest is FICA/Medicare (Federal Insurance Contributions Act), also referred to as Social Security or SSI, or in another context as the self-employment tax. Employers and employees split these taxes; employers can deduct their half as an expense. Each half is 7.65%, and together they add up to 15.3%. ICs are responsible for the entire amount, although half of it is treated as a deductible expense. There is no difference in sole proprietor and corporate treatment.

Workman's comp is technically not required for a sole proprietor (depending on the state, a corporate officer may also be exempt), but if you hire other employees, it is an absolute requirement. The hospital may require it or some other form of accident insurance. I have also read recommendations that ICs should carry workman's comp, regardless of the requirements. It costs perhaps 2% of gross payroll, so it is up to your judgment. Rules also vary quite a bit from state to state.

Unemployment insurance has a state and federal component and also accounts for about 2% of payroll. It is optional for a sole proprietor and usually a corporate officer, but not for their employees. I can't think of a good reason to pay this, and you won't be eligible for benefits anyway. It is also a cost advantage you have over an agency (you could reduce your bill rate by 2% for example to be more competitive).

The easiest way to reduce all taxes is by seeking out and taking all available legitimate expense deductions. Don't spend money just to save on taxes; that is just foolish—he more you spend the more you save theory. Deductions that a travel nurse IC should consider are meals and incidentals from Publication 1542, housing away from your tax home (leveraged with Publication 1542 schedules if you are a corporation), all travel between your tax home and the facility (if an overnight stay) at 37.5 cents a mile (or actual airfare/other costs if higher), commute miles between temporary housing and the hospital, licenses, education R/T profession, certifications, cell phones. Perhaps you have to hire people to maintain your home while you are away. Anything business related should be considered, including lawyer, CPA, other consultant fees, books about business, incorporation and maintenance costs, and bank fees.

Business structure directly impacts payroll taxes. So corporation can pass through some of their profits to their owners without being subject to payroll taxes. (See Business entities FAQ.) C corps may likewise be able to figure out a scheme to do this. Be careful and get good advice, though; bonuses for officers or employees are usually considered reportable wages. Dividends to shareholders, while not subject to payroll taxes, are subject to both corporate income tax *and* personal income tax (double taxation).

In Conclusion

This is only a tip of the iceberg when it comes to the world of independent contracting. This, along with other resources including the IRS website, small business associations, and discussion boards on independent contracting or nursing entrepreneurship, will have you headed down the road to success.

~*~

Big thanks to Ned for allowing me to use portions of his website for some content in this chapter. Ned, RN, is the host of the Independent Contractors forum at: http://forums.delphiforums.com/ICNurse/, a forum that allows independent nurses to network, ask questions, and give advice to other independent nurses and those who wish to become independent contractors in the nursing or the broader healthcare community.

Other aspects of this chapter were written from my personal experience of being a sole proprietor of an eBook publishing company, travel nursing informational site, and being partial owner in an Internet Service Providership, which was classified as an S-Corp along with my husband's experience in both C-Corporations and Limited Liability Corporations.

Although a business plan and marketing plan are not set in stone must-haves, I do believe that it is a great way to plan out what you are trying to accomplish and have available if someone ever questions the validity of your company.

Chapter Thirteen

What About Homeschooling?

For years I thought that I couldn't do travel nursing because my son was in public school and that I needed to give him a stable environment in which to live. I planned on going into travel nursing the minute he graduated. That was until April 2003.

My son's school informed me that my child had figured out that if he went to this in-school suspension program, he could do his schoolwork in another classroom without all the kids who called him names and picked on him unmercifully. Kids are just cruel in junior high school, and if you don't conform to their idea of what a "cool" teenager is.

The counselor told me, "I just don't know what I'm going to do with your son next year." I looked at my husband, who shrugged, and then I turned to the school counselor and advised him that I didn't think that he was going to have to worry about my son next year.

My bachelor's degree actually is not in nursing; it's in secondary science education. After we went home, I informed my husband that I believed that it was time to hit the road. If they didn't know what to do with him, I didn't see where it would harm my child to be on the road fulltime in an "unstable" environment when he could learn things all over the United States.

I had a teacher's certificate at one time (lapsed when I went into nursing), and I didn't see where the school system was doing a better job than I could do at home. My suspicions were confirmed when I did his diagnostic testing and found that my 7th grader was actually functioning at a 3rd to 4th grade level. That made me a real believer in the Individual Educational Program (IEP) that schools have now set forth.

Okay, off of my soap-box and back into the real world of homeschooling! The decision was easy for me, since I had an educational degree background. After this chapter, you will have the knowledge to make an informed decision on whether or not homeschooling is right for you and your children, as well as what alternatives you have.

Exactly What Is Homeschooling?

Homeschooling is getting out the books every morning and doing lessons in math, science, history, grammar, and literature. Homeschooling is taking field trips. Homeschooling is running around in your pajama's doing algebra. Homeschooling is many different things that all surround the idea of teaching your children at home.

First is the traditional style of homeschooling. This follows the traditional way of doing schoolwork. With this style, you find books that are geared towards the age and grade of your child and you have traditional reading, worksheets, and then tests. There are several curriculums that you can use for this style, including Alpha Omega Lifepacs (which use workbooks) or textbooks through Abeka Publishing or Bob Jones Publishing, which are Christian- based curriculums. I also found some secular programs at www.myeducationathome.com. I am not familiar with the company or all the textbooks, but I was familiar with some of the textbooks that were in the packets.

Another great source is to find out what the schools do with their old books. I found a gold mine of used school books in Oklahoma City. I also purchased a book with a plethora of resources called, "The Complete Home Learning Source Book." Check with your local homeschool association and find out when and where the next book fair is going to be. You can also get an idea of what other parents are using before you set out on your travel nursing adventure.

Computer learning is next on the list. Through one program called "Switched On Schoolhouse" or the "Robinson Curriculum," you install the program onto your computer and your child's computer and you have control over the student's curriculum. This is a great way to do things for some children and teachers alike. The lessons are automatically graded, and learning is on an interactive level.

Computer learning can also be accomplished with some programs online in which you enroll your child in a school, and they take classes online with teachers and tests through the Internet. This is a great option for the parent who is uneasy about attempting to teach their child at home.

Unit studies are very popular also. This is where you teach your children all subjects that are on one subject (this is confusing and needs to be reworded). This can be very useful as a traveling nurse, because you can do unit studies on the state in which you are traveling as well as the surrounding states. Children are taught math, as in how much is needed to purchase groceries; history through the state sites; biology through seeing what grows in that area and what type of energy is most common there, and are there any windmills or hydro plants? You can view guides for unit studies at: www.homeschoolunitstudies.com and www.homeschoollearning.com. By doing a search online you can find free unit study guides.

The new out-of-the-box type of homeschooling is called "un-schooling." This is where the children learn from day-to-day events. No, this does not mean that they sit and watch television and play video games all day, but things are learned from experiences. Parents will often spend time going through the newspaper with their children and learning what is going on in the world and why things are happening the way they are. Math is learned from figuring out how much things cost, how to budget, and other word problems. Science is learned by exploring a park and checking out all the leaves and grasses and attempting to identify what kind of things are in the environment. No tests are done, but the children learn by experience. I think this is a great way of learning for travel nurses to incorporate at least part-time, since we travel so much and see so many different things and live in so many different cultures.

All these curriculums can be found by doing a search online, contacting the publishing houses, and on eBay. If you are interested in looking at sources in your community, find your local homeschool association and ask for their help in finding homeschool materials. Materials can also be found at general bookstores. Even Borders, Barnes and Noble, and Hastings can special order books for you.

Personally, I buy my books online at PennywiseLearning.com or on eBay. After my son had completed all his material on another sheet of paper or in his notebook, I then sold the material as used on eBay and recovered at least half of the money that I had spent to get the books.

What About State Laws?

Laws are different in each state. As a traveling nurse, you primarily have to go by what your home state laws are, but there are certain situations when you will have to abide by the state laws to which you are assigned.

For instance, in Mississippi they have a law that states that all recreational vehicle parks have to have documentation that your child, who is running around during the day, actually is homeschooled. For this, I just gave the park manager a copy of the affidavit that I had filled out for my home state, affirming that my child was homeschooled. This may also mean getting a letter from the school district in states that require you to keep in touch with the school district.

When we were in Tennessee, we didn't have to have a letter for the apartment complex, but we did have to have a letter for my 17-year-old's place of employment from the school board, stating that our son was enrolled in homeschool. To accomplish this, I wrote a letter of intent to the school board here and sent them verification of my qualifications to teach, and they sent me a letter for my son's employer that stated he was in homeschool. It was then that I realized that in some states you must have a copy of your bachelor's degree in order to teach high school.

Why did I have to go through all of this? Because in different states you have different age requirements on how long your children must attend school. Although we were okay with our home state of Idaho, we still had to comply with some of the state requirements because of housing and employment. There are other states that we have been in (Oklahoma, Florida, California, and Iowa) where we were not required to do anything special related to our home residence, since it was not in those states. If there is a problem, someone will tell you that until that time it is usually best just to cruise through your assignment following your home state's rules.

Finding out the laws in each state is not as difficult as you would think; all you need to do is bookmark on your computer www.hslda.org. If you do not have a computer, the information can also be found through that state's department of education or local school district.

Some of the state laws are very restrictive and some are not so restrictive. For example, in Idaho the only rules are that if your child is between the ages of 7 years and 15 you must have some kind of alternative educational program. That means that once children are 16 they can "drop out" of school, although it is not necessarily advised. Other less restrictive states that I have been in are Texas and Oklahoma.

Medium restrictive states that I have been in include Arizona, California, and Mississippi. These states require such things as filing an annual affidavit or letter of intent, maintaining attendance records, and requiring basic subjects such as math, science, history, grammar, and literature. Tennessee also requires that you must have a college education to teach high school and that your child has to attend school until they are 18.

Other more restrictive states require you to have more extensive subjects, such as algebra, geometry, physics and chemistry, along with documentation of the hours spent in school, days spent in school, maintaining accurate records, and taking state- wide standardized tests.

Driving Me Crazy

Literally, for a homeschooled child of a traveling nurse, I was literally nuts by the time we wove our way through all the legal mumble jumble, but we made it.

Driver's education at our house was done by the "principal"—i.e. Dad! If you are located in a heavily populated area, I would suggest that you find a good driving school. If you are in a rural area, good old country roads that are unpopulated provide a good start. Talk to other nurses to see if someone has a place out in the country for a "feel" of what it is like to drive for the first time. Of course this is only done after your child has a learning permit.

Getting the learning permit—*that* was what drove me crazy with all these state rules. It is always best to have your child take the test in the state in which you are a resident, but if you are across the country and you think that your child is ready, then it can be done in some states. The key to this is that hopefully you are in a state in which your son/daughter can be a resident of that state, and you do not have to be. This is easily accomplished if your child has some kind of employment. For instance, at the time we still had the RV and my son worked for the campground part-time. It wasn't much, but it did give him a paycheck. We used a national bank, separate from our bank, and used his address as the assignment address. Sonny has a job and a bank account, now he can pass for a resident—well, at least in some states.

There are other states in which the parents also have to have a driver's license in that state. Although not advisable, but if need be, your spouse can get a driver's license in the new state, but do not ever get your driver's license in another state, because then you are going to have trouble with the Internal Revenue Service in establishing a tax home. It's not going to look good with your spouse being a resident of another state, but it is just one option to consider.

As previously stated, if at all possible find a local driving school for your child; if one can not be found, there are lots of driver's programs online, such as the one found at www.driversed.com. After completing the program, your child will receive a certificate of completion, which is approved by almost all the states (verify before you begin if you wish). It is just a great course that I would recommend to anybody homeschooling their child.

Also, contact your insurance agency and see if they have programs available. We watched a movie and filled out a driving log to receive a discount on our insurance; you can also have your child take the SAT or ACT test and get a reduced "good student" rate. In fact, we kept a travel log for a while after my son completed his regular program in case we needed to prove how many hours he had behind the wheel.

One of the funniest experiences with this whole deal is when we moved assignments, my son went to apply for his regular permit instead of a learner's permit and they wanted to know if he had any experience with a certified driving instructor. Of course he hadn't, but we had made a trip between assignments back home so he had driven most of the way from Iowa home to Idaho and to Florida. Over 3000 miles and none of it counted because he wasn't with a certified driving instructor.

What About Socialization?

You know what is funny about people who ask this question? They will also tell you about the terrible things that happened at Columbine High School, the Red Lake shootings, and all the teens that are arrested at school for having guns in their possession. Why did all these bad things happen at school? Because the majority of teens think that to be cool you have to knock someone else's "coolness" down. Unless your child is perfect, chances are they are being teased or bullied at school by someone. That is what I call "great socialization"!

At one of the RV parks we were in the owner and manager said that the children were not allowed to use the recreational equipment on the weekends when other children were there, but they had found that the homeschooled children were much better behaved and they could go over anytime if it was just them. Several times I had people come to my trailer and ask if "the boy over there is your son?" After answering "Yes," they would proceed to tell me what good things my son had done and then asked, "Is he homeschooled?" I don't know what other proof you need, but my personal experience is that people can tell by your child's behavior that they are homeschooled.

Yes, I believe that our children need to be around other children of the same age, but with the proper influence. After getting settled into an area we start the search for a church that has a good group of teenagers. I am a member of the Nazarene Church, and my husband was born and raised Baptist; therefore, we tend to stick to one of those two denominations, but there was one assignment in which we were Lutherans, related to the fact that that is where the best group of teenagers was for our son to be social with.

Other than church groups, there are many other groups such as Boy Scouts, Girl Scouts, and Explorer Groups. Look for groups such as a bowling league, baseball league, basketball league, or the YMCA. The local Chamber of Commerce or parks and recreation departments at the city should be able to help you in choosing a place for your child to interact with other children. Also, look for information through the local homeschool association.

From A Child

As a writing assignment, I asked Kalen what he would like to tell others about his life as the son of a fulltime traveling nurse, and this is what he had to say.

"I love traveling with my parents because I get to see so many exciting places. When I was in Arizona, I got to see the Grand Canyon, and I have been to an old gold mine. I got to go to the London Bridge on several occasions. In 2001, my family and I went several times to Chase Stadium, which was known back then as Bank One Ballpark, in Phoenix to see the Diamondbacks play. This is also the year that the won the World Series.

When I was in California, I got to do several things including learning a little Spanish, going to Monterey to go deep sea fishing in the Pacific Ocean, and I even got to experience my first earthquake.

When we went to Iowa, I got my first job at a restaurant near the lake. Mom and I also got to go to the see the scene of the crash where Buddy Holly, the Big Bopper, and Ritchie Valens passed away, which is now known as the day that the music died.

When I went to Oklahoma, I was in Oklahoma City. I got to go to the Oklahoma Bombing site. Although I was living in Oklahoma at the time of the bombing, I don't remember much of it, so it was great to learn about something that happened while I was an Okie. In Tulsa we went to see the Tulsa Drillers, which is a AAA baseball team. I met a few friends there also. We also went to Tulsa to get my 16th birthday present, a 1985 Ford Mustang Convertible in which my uncle painted for me.

Our fifth assignment was in Mississippi. I got to go to Corinth where the north and south train route met with the east to west train at the crossroads. I got to visit several battlefields, but the most memorable one was the site of the Battle of Shiloh.

Next we went to Florida. While I was there, I worked for a local newspaper and then started my fast food career. Hurricane Wilma came to visit us, and that was a totally different experience for me! There was so much devastation in Florida that I can't imagine what it was like for those who were in Hurricane Katrina.

Unfortunately my mustang didn't make it out of Florida. When I was driving from Fort Lauderdale, Florida, to Nashville, Tennessee, the engine gave it up on the side of the road. I will just have to wait until the next assignment to think about another vehicle.

Right now I'm in Tennessee. I have made a great career choice here. I love my fast food job, and have even been recommended for a managerial position when I turn 18 years old. I have always wanted to be a police officer, but I am currently thinking about going into restaurant management instead.

Although I have had some great adventures over the last three years, there have been some drawbacks. Seems like every time that I get settled into a job and a new store, then it's time to move again. I have a long list of friends, but I don't see them. Most of my friends don't come from school, but from the church youth groups that I attend while on the road. I also miss my friend in my old hometown of Lake Havasu City, Arizona.

I also met my girlfriend on the road through the internet. I haven't got to meet her yet, but my mom says that she is going to take an assignment in Washington this next year so that we can meet "in reality." This may seem strange to some teens, but hey, my mom and step-dad met that away! We have been chatting on the phone and computer for almost two years now.

I have learned so much more traveling than I ever could learn in a classroom. I would definitely recommend nurses taking their children with them if at all possible. I love my life on the road! Thanks, Mom!"

In Conclusion

No, homeschooling is not for every parent on the road, but I have had several nurses ask me exactly how I homeschool my child, how I started out, and the benefits that I have found since we're on the road fulltime.

Yes, there are other ways to provide school for children while on the road, such as switching assignments in the middle of semesters at Christmas break and during summer break. You can get in three good assignments this way. Others that I know take a nine-month assignment during the school year and then take a summer assignment somewhere in the cooler north or on the beach. Other parents choose to stay within a few hundred miles of their families, and their families stay at home. There is no *one* right or wrong way to school your child while on the road. You have to do what is most comfortable for you and your family.

For those of you who choose to homeschool, the freedom of learning live historical facts is worth "dragging" your children around the United States. I have absolutely no doubt that it makes them better students for the future, and I hope that this chapter will give you the motivation that you need to make that leap into the future of homeschooling.

Chapter Fourteen

Taking Your Home with You on Assignment

Making The Decision To Travel In An RV

Whether I was in Oklahoma, Mississippi, California or Iowa, I have always had the same accommodation—a thirty-six foot travel trailer. Not exactly luxurious accommodations, but at least I didn't have to pack and unpack every three to six months. No, this lifestyle is not for everyone, but for me and my family it was just perfect.

It all started after my first assignment. Moving into the apartment in Phoenix was okay for the three of us, until we went to move out. Our home was two hundred miles away from the assignment and we found ourselves taking more and more stuff down each time we returned to the Phoenix apartment from our home in Lake Havasu City, Arizona.

After taking two trips with a U-Haul trailer to get everything back, we decided that we didn't adjust very well to keeping it downsized at the apartment. With the three of us, we needed to either buy a bigger permanent hauling trailer or look at a travel trailer.

Off to California I went, while my son and husband stayed back in Arizona to gather up some loose ends before joining me. I was by myself for one month, living in a motel room, since housing was scarce related to seasonal workers.

After the family joined me, we moved into a larger motel suite, but that quickly became too close for comfort, hence the search for the alternative of a recreational vehicle (RV).

What Type To Look For

What exactly people are looking for in an RV and their needs are so diverse that companies have been expanding their floor plans on a yearly basis. We started our hunt for an RV by visiting as many dealers as we could find in central California. When you go, be sure to also ask about any RV shows that might be coming up in the area.

After you have been to a few dealers, make a list of exactly what you want in an RV. Also, when you are out browsing, look at several different types of RVs. Most full-timers are either in a Class A Motorhome, Class C Motorhome, Travel Trailer or 5th Wheel.

The least expensive of these options is a travel trailer. A good one will average $15K to $30K, depending on size. If you are full-timing by yourself, you might consider one that is 25 ft. in length. If there are two of you, I would consider a 30=ft model. If you have children, look at one of the bigger ones at 35-39ft., with a bunk system in the back.

Thirty-six feet seemed to be just right for our family of three. It had two bedrooms; therefore, everyone still had some sense of private space. I know of another traveler who has a four-bunk system, in which he and his wife travel with their four children.

Your next option, price-wise, would be a fifth wheel. These are generally priced from $30K to $80K on the new market. According to a friend of mind, those are much easier to handle than a bumper-pulled travel trailer and easier to hook/unhook from your vehicle. Unfortunately, my truck has a permanent tonneau cover on it; therefore, we are unable to pull a 5th wheel.

In Arkansas I came across a travel nurse who was living in a Class C Motorhome. Those are the smaller Motorhomes that are usually easily recognized by the over-the-cab bed or storage.

The cost of these run on the average $60K to $100K. Being that they are smaller, they are most often looked at by a first timer or female who isn't comfortable with the idea of owning or driving a larger "bus"-sized vehicle. They come in many variations now, including with slide-out and storage compartments instead of a bed over-the-cab.

This type of home might be looked at by a couple of a family of four, with the option of the over-cab-queen size bed for the parents and twin beds in the back for the children. I could definitely picture myself in one of these if I were a single female. Instead of having to get out for sleeping or using the restroom while on the road, you can just pull over and go to the back and leave the doors locked.

The largest and most expensive option would be a Class A Motorhome, which are the ones that are "bus"-sized. These range in price from $80K to over a million dollars.

Nice and spacious, they are definitely homes-away-from-home! Your gasoline Class As are the least expensive options, but they also have the lowest resale value. The diesel Class As are more expensive, but they hold more of their value when it comes time for a resale.

Coming in a wide variety, many are from 35 ft/ to 40 ft. on the average; these babies come packed not only with a kitchen sink, but also a dishwasher as an option. After taking a tour of a factory in Iowa, I ventured into an RV that not only had a flat screen television, but also a complete entertainment system, including a fireplace. Now *that* is what I call entertainment!

Basic Buying Guide

Take a look at many floor plans. Where are the beds and the kitchen? We have found, in buying a travel trailer, that it is easier when stopping along the way if the bed is in the back. This way you can load up the kitchen/living area in the front of the trailer, with the bath in the middle. This way you can have all the extra weight in the front and you don't have to load and unload all the extras every time. All that is required is to open up the back door and crawl into the bed.

If you have a motorhome, make sure that you have a path from the front of the rig to the back where your bed is, or when on the road use the fold-out couch in the front of the coach and store all the extra stuff in the back. This, of course, will all depend on how many "extra" goodies you have along with you. We carried an extra outdoor table and chairs, plus at one time I had my outdoor barrel pond. The less you carry, the better off you are, but as any traveler can tell you, that is always easier said than done.

With any travel trailer or 5th wheel, the first thing you need to know is how much weight your tow vehicle can handle. In your operator's guide you will find the towing capacity. Tell the dealer, the first thing, what type of vehicle you are using for a tow vehicle, what type of tow package (extra transmission cooler and gauges), and any special items you might have on the vehicle that would effect its towing capacity. For example, our truck will pull 9500 lbs, we have an external and internal transmission cooler, extra transmission gauges, and air suspension.

Once you know the amount that your vehicle can pull, you want to look for a trailer that is about 70% of that weight. Therefore, the trailer that I would be looking for would be approximately 6650 lbs. Once you have added all your living supplies, the trailer should weight no more than 80% of your towing capacity. If, for some reason, you go over your 100% towing capacity and you get into an accident, you have a good chance of being liable, due to the fact that your weight limit exceeds what your vehicle can handle.

Make sure that you have the proper hitch, also. You not only need the proper size ball hitch, but you need the appropriate weight distribution bar, anti-sway bar, and get the best brake control system that you can afford. Skimping on these details can make a big difference if you get into high winds, going up and down steep grades, or in case you need to make an emergency stop.

A big thing for full-timers is storage! Make sure that you have enough storage. This is where the motorhomes have a great advantage over a travel trailer. The "basement" storage is a great plus. There is also more closet space in the motorhomes than in a travel trailer on the average; although I have been in a few 5th wheels that have quite a bit of closet space. If you have a handyman around, an option for a travel trailer would be to convert a bunk system in a travel trailer to more closet space. One trailer I looked at last year in a home show had a small slide- out in the back where the kids had their own couch and entertainment center, along with fold up bunks. In my situation, it would be so easy to take out the bunks and make a closet out of that and use the small slide-out for an office space. When we were looking at toy-haulers once, a dealer told us about a full timer who couldn't find exactly what she needed, so she took an empty trailer and put in her own furniture to make a home-on-wheels. In other words, use your imagination when you go shopping!

A few other things to consider when shopping are the bedroom and bathroom. Lie on the bed and see how it feels. Some aren't the most comfortable beds, but can be made more manageable by putting one of those space-age technology types of foam mattresses over it. In the last few years I have seen more and more motorhomes with the sleep number bed system as an option. You can also purchase a sleep number bed mattress system at your local camping supply store.

Sit on the commode and see if there is enough leg and arm space. The last few years I have seen more and more RVs with the optional shower on one side and the commode on the other side. What size shower and/or tub do you need? We were very lucky in the fact that we had a full-size tub. There wasn't too much difference between the tub size in my permanent home and my RV. Some have half-tubs and some just have the shower. This last year I even saw one that had a whirlpool tub in it, although that motorhome was a little more expensive than I could afford at $350K.

Also, look at what type of electrical system it has. The standard RV has either 30 amp or 50 amp, unless you get a gigantic motorhome, which may require 100 amp. With a 30 amp vehicle you might find yourself turning off the air conditioner while you run the microwave or blow-dry your hair. Usually, with a 50 amp, you don't have to worry about that. Also, it will make a big difference if you have one or two air conditioning units. With the RVs that have two air conditioning units, you will need a 50 amp or an upgraded electrical system that can handle all of the power needs.

What Options To Look For

In the beginning of the RV building world there were only two or three floor plans and styles that you could choose from, but now the options are almost endless.

In the travel trailer world you can find trailers with garages, trailers that have "toy boxes" for your motorcycles or golf cart, ones with slide-outs, and trailers with utility closets in the back.

In Arizona and Southern California, the toy haulers are quite common. Not only do people haul around their dune buggies and four wheelers, but golf carts and small electric cars. With gas prices soaring ever so high, I have often thought about getting a toy box and an electric car.

The smaller garages at the back would also be nice for a full-timer. You could store things that you might use seasonally or keep your bikes locked up. The other day we saw an RV with a small storage area in the whole back of the trailer that opened up and you could hang items like your hoses, utility equipment, and miscellaneous hardware in there.

Other options that you may look for in the kitchen are a full-size or four-door refrigerator and freezer with an ice-maker. These are great and can be found in a lot of the newer motorhomes. Also, in the kitchens of the newer motorhomes you might find a dishwasher or a trash compactor.

In many of the 5th wheels and motorhomes you might find a combination washer and dryer. Although these are very small, they are great to use for everyday clothes. You will probably still want to use the bigger machines at the laundromat for your bigger items, such as towels and linens.

In the living room area you can look for such options as an electric fireplace, entertainment center, computer center and satellite dish. Satellite dishes also come in many types, from just plain old television to ones that will also help you get onto the Internet and even track while moving (this will be discussed later on in more depth).

To make traveling and maneuvering easier you can find motorhomes with a navigational system and cameras in the back of the rig to assist you in backing up. After you have had either of these for very long you will wonder how you ever lived without them! I can't imagine going anywhere without my navigational system.

Motorhomes usually come with some kind of basement storage. This is the one major advantage to having a larger motorhome; there is a lot more storage for full-timers! There is even one company who not only makes a basement, but also has an upstairs. That's right, a set of stairs leads you to the top of the RV where there is a patio set up with grill, tables, chairs, and an umbrella. Of course you would want to take the umbrella down while you're going down the road. Ha!

There are many, many other options that you can have. What you have to decide is which options are worth the money for you and your family.

Internet Access While On The Road

There are several ways to do this. Most of the RV parks now have a computer station in which there is a phone line that you can plug into for dial-up Internet. Sometimes there is a small fee or time limit on this service, but it is available. You may just want to get a phone and have dialup service that way.

Another option is through your cell phone. For about $20, you can purchase a cable that will connect your cell phone to your computer through the USB port. After purchasing a dialup program for another $20, you can then use your phone. Check with your cell phone carrier about charges for this service. Some companies take air time out of your minutes, while others will let you use it unlimited for a set price.

Wireless cards are also an option. These cards are offered through cell phone companies and are like a wireless system that you plug into the network port on your laptop. In the bigger cities you can have up to broadband speeds with these systems; although the current price is about $80/month.

Wireless systems at campgrounds are also an up and coming thing. Some campgrounds charge for this service, but the ones I have frequented had no extra charge for this service. Once at the campground, search for wireless networks, find the park network and take off at racing speeds. You may have to have a password from the front office if it is a secure network. In fact, just recently the Good Sam's Club has contracted with a network carrier to provide wireless to all of its campgrounds.

For your own personal broadband network you can also do the satellite Internet. There are three types that you can get. The first is a dish that is set up on a tripod. Every time you go to a new place, you set up the tripod and dish, aim the satellite, and you're off and running. The first couple of times you try it can be frustrating, but after much perseverance, you can do it! After my husband sets ours up, I can shoot it within five to ten minutes now.

Another system is on top of the rig, and you still have to manually adjust it every time. This really isn't too bad if you are moving only once every three to six months and can be easily figured out as with the tripod system. The disadvantage to this is that you have to make sure that your rig is perfectly level or you won't be able to find the satellite connection.

The least work that you will have to do is with an automatic satellite, but it is much more expensive than the first two. In fact, a few years ago I paid $1,500 for my system on the tripod, while a friend of mine paid $5,000 for her automatic one on top of the rig. It seems like she has more trouble with her system than I have with my system, and every time there is a problem she has to take her rig into the dealer to have the satellite worked on, where ours is much more easily repaired, being that it is not connected to the rig. The system that you choose will depend on how computer savvy you are.

The drawback from having a system like mine is that you either have to be certified to aim the satellite or hire a certified installer to come out and aim the dish every time you move. I would recommend taking the class so you can aim your own dish, like I did.

In Conclusion

The mobile lifestyle is one that can be very rewarding if you hate packing and unpacking every few months. If you keep your traveling goodies to a minimum, your home can easily be unhooked from the park and moved in a just a few short hours.

The article in my newsletter that this chapter was based upon was written last year while I was on assignment in Iowa. My family and I loved our trailer, but on the way to Florida we learned that rain and 18-wheelers who pass you while going downhill don't mix. After our little fishtailing episode, the frame was so bent up that it slid into the tires once we got to Kansas City, leaving us "homeless" in Missouri. We bought the little black cargo trailer to pack all the stuff that we had in the travel trailer, and currently take the company apartment.

We sure miss our little home of two years, but just haven't found the right one to continue our adventures on the road in an RV. I guess the thing I miss most is going camping on the way to assignments in the different state parks. Take your time, enjoy the mobile life in an RV, and don't be afraid to "rough it" at the state parks on the road. There are plenty of them, and they are less expensive than camping out in a RV park all the time. Take it easy, enjoy nature and the deer in the morning when you're having coffee.

Chapter Fifteen

Politics In Travel Nursing

Although most of us go into travel nursing to get out of the hospital politics, there are a few things that affect travel nursing in a political fashion.

Three of the most recent developments include: JCAHO accreditation of healthcare staffing agencies, the Nursing Compact, and the Performance Based Development System (PBDS). This chapter will explore these new elements of travel nursing and how they will affect your career as a travel nurse.

JCAHO

The Joint Commission on Accreditation of Healthcare Organizations (JCAHO) has recently set new standards for healthcare staffing agencies. This new certification process will mean big changes in the travel-nursing field. What does this means for staffing companies? New standards have been placed on the travel-staffing companies and on travel nurses. The staffing companies will have to clearly define the company leadership hierarchy.

The hierarchy of the travel company will include the administrator, director of nursing services, recruiters, and traveling nurses. The recruiter most likely will have a regional supervisor, an account manager, or a recruiting manager. Also in the mix will be the accountant, payroll supervisor, information systems technician, human resources, and a housing supervisor. The new JCAHO standards will mean that travelers have to get used to the formal processes, but it will also prevent finger-pointing at travelers and in effect will assist in the protection of the travel nurse's license.

The administrator, nursing director, accountant or chief financial officer will also be in charge of the development and monitoring of an annual budget. This budget will include costs of certifications, cost of management, cost of the nurses, costs of the benefits, and how that amount compares with the accounts receivable through the hospital bill rate. Where is this going to lead?

With the implementation of JCAHO certifications, the initial cost of owning a staffing company just increased. This cost is proportionate to national versus regional coverage and the overall size of the company. The cost of JCAHO certification is determined by the number of branch offices that the staffing company is operating. Although the initial cost may be in the thousands of dollars, the efficiencies that certification puts in place increases the effectiveness that keep both hospital and travelers happier in the long run. Staffing companies have found that since the implementation of JCAHO standards, more contracts from hospitals have been offered to the staffing companies; therefore, the jobs available to nurses have increased.

Most certainly, not all staffing companies will be able to survive all these costs; therefore, companies either will have to do more subcontracting through companies which can afford the JCAHO certification or the smaller companies will be forced to comply with JCAHO standards through subcontracting to JCAHO certified firms; either way, eventually all firms will have to be JCAHO compliant.

With the money crunch that is put on smaller companies, some travel nurses believe that this will lead to Cross Country Trav Corp, Intelistaf, and AMN Healthcare will become the Walmart, Kmart, and Target of travel companies, with the smaller companies like Nursing Options and All Health Staffing fighting to keep alive. Nurses know that they get better service with the smaller companies, but we also know that jobs with these smaller companies are few.

A top priority addressed by the JCAHO certification team is a code of ethics—a code that says the staffing office will take every precaution to provide a work environment that is free of harassment, treats everyone equally, and in short treats people like human beings.

As a nurse, I expect companies to treat me like a name, and not a number. Along with treating me as a name, also please have the decency to call nurses by the name that they wish to be called. Not every nurse goes by their given "first name." Since 9-11-2001, first names have become more of a security issue. You can put my first given name on my paycheck and office IRS documents, but when I call the office I expect you to call me by my middle name, which I have gone by for over twenty-five years. It totally amazed me when I called the larger company that I traveled with for over a year and they couldn't find me in their system under the name that I go by, but they found me in the system by my social security number. I was definitely just a number, and not a name to everyone else but my recruiter.

Respect and ethics have other faces, including sticking with your nurses when the times get tough. Nurses must respect their agencies to be truthful and honest in every situation. Nurses must have ethics and professionalism every day on the job, and the expectations should also be there for the staffing agencies.

Another issue addressed by JCAHO pertains to getting business through other unfair means, including contract discrepancies, making your travel assignment your permanent assignment, and other conflicts between the hospital and the nurse. JCAHO now mandates that travelers be protected in their contracts, particularly for professional liability insurance, floating, orientation, and incident or complaint reporting. Contract discrepancies can include anything from unsuitable housing to pay being contracted as one thing and paid at another rate, and a pay rate that is verbally agreed upon, then changed in the written contract.

Conflicts can also occur when a nurse wants to continue on as a permanent staffing member instead of as contracted staff. Some companies put a six-month to one year clause in there that says you cannot go from travel to permanent after a certain period of time. Staffing companies must have a plan to deal with the above situations, and any others of the like that come up. When there are problems with the nurse's performance, the hospital has a right to terminate that contract, but there is usually a conflict between how much the employee is penalized monetarily for housing and travel. If the employee feels that they were wrongfully terminated, they have the problem of a wrongful contract termination. There must be a plan of action to assist with this conflict, which includes incident reporting that JCAHO requires from the hospital.

There are always two sides to every story, and conflicts can only be solved through a structured plan and the assistance of mediation, if needed. Conflicts and problems do not always occur Monday through Friday, 9am to 5pm. There must be a twenty-four- hour support telephone line available. The problems that do occur must be promptly solved. The longer the problem lingers, the greater the problem becomes.

The next big issue is that of quality nursing care. Quality must be assured by skills checklists, orientation skills checked off, and standard safety proficiency. Safety issues are addressed initially with the use of skills checklists, which are completed by the nurse upon application for the position. If a hospital reports that clinically a nurse is not able to perform as stated, then it is the agency's job to work with the nurse to either find different placement or help the nurse to obtain the credentials. These skills checklists must also be updated every year.

Another aspect of JCAHO standards is the issue of quality assurance and making sure that the credentials and experience correlate to the work history record. For example, if the nurse says that she knows about Swan-Ganz arterial lines, wouldn't it make sense that she must have worked in critical care? Standard safety issues, including blood borne pathogens, fire safety, back safety, and safely getting from the hospital parking lot to your floor and back at the end of your shift are also things that need to be addressed in orientation and yearly educational programs. There are rules now about required yearly continuing education, which will hopefully eliminate repeat paper work at your assignment.

A big safety issue that is a prominent concern is nurse-to-patient ratios. It is the travel nurse's responsibility to assure that they are not being put into an unsafe situation, during the interview with the hospital. It is the staffing agency's responsibility to stand behind the nurse with these staffing issues. This is accomplished by the new JCAHO complaint reporting laws. If the nurse-to-patient ratio is not as stated in the interview, then the staffing company and nurse need to do some conflict resolvement with the hospital's management team.

Evaluations from supervisors are also an important tool in safety and quality of care. These evaluations are used to determine if the job is really going as well or as bad as the travel nurse states it is. Then again, we have to remember that there are two sides to every story, but usually if things are bad, things are bad on both sides, and conflict mediation may be needed to continue quality nursing care.

JCAHO standards also involve continuing education. Continuing education, as well as experience, is what makes a good nurse even better. Education must also be provided for age specific aspects, patient confidentiality, HIPPA Privacy Compliance, Infection Control, and how to help the patients who have been involved in a domestic abusive situation. This is most often correlated in the orientation process and quality of care issues that were mentioned above. A nurse's skills must be kept up-to-date and new education opportunities taken advantage of in the area of expertise.

When these quality measures become issues, then a staffing company must have an organized approach to improve the nurse's performance. This can be done through educational opportunities and other opportunities for improvement. If required, verbal warnings, written warnings, and termination may be inevitable if these opportunities are not taken advantage of. If there is a conflict between what is stated on paper and what the nurse's performance is, the hospital has the responsibility to report it to the staffing agency. What was the problem? What attempts were made to solve the problem? What was the outcome? What is the percentage of travel nurses that stay with the staffing company? Why did the travel nurse leave the staffing company? Were their problems with the company, or just problems related to location or benefits?

All this information provided by the hospital, the nurse, and other information from the staffing company pertaining to the employment of the nurse must be kept in a secure and confidential environment. A plan must be in place in order to maintain confidential information about the hospital that is being staffed also.

Along with all of this goes the process for maintaining continuity of information. The records of each nurse must be safeguarded. The information must be available to the nurse, if needed, for other staffing opportunities. Profiles only need to be submitted upon approval of the nurse. Profiles must not be lost within the system! I had a situation where I was transferring to a different office. One week after I had moved, my file mysteriously disappeared from the office. Was my information in a safe and confidential place?

Ummmm... Another nurse told me the same type of story with the same company. Maybe, with the new JCAHO certifications and regulations, this problem will not continue to occur. Files won't get lost and employees won't get lost in the system.

What is the future of travel nursing? Many travelers that I have talked to have raised concerns that the staffing agencies will have to be JCAHO certified in order to place nurses in JCAHO certified hospitals; however, the cost of this certification will usually increase the bill rate to the hospital, so pay should remain proportionate. The agency will have to renew their certification every two years. Travel nurses should be accountable for themselves and have personal quality control and ethics; those who are in it for the money and not concerned about patient care are the ones whom this will affect the most. Over all travel nurses are quality nurses, who have great expectations placed on them.

I was recently discussing this with Greg Allen, president of Cirrus Medical Staffing, and he feels that many of the nurses may become discouraged because of all the paperwork required to remain a traveler, since their company is JCAHO certified. All updates must occur on a bi-yearly basis. Though travelers are used to the standard licensure, certification and medical updates yearly, they will now have to update other tests, such as medication tests, age competency tests, abbreviation standards, various required continuing education requirements, and the list will continue to grow as JCAHO certification becomes the standard for staffing firms and other safety issues are identified. The best way to handle this is to request copies or make copies of all required paperwork and keep for yourself at all times. This will make switching companies much easier when needed.

Another impact may be that the travelers must become more open to and willing to float to other units, which hospitals will be forced to show evidence of an appropriate orientation of another similar unit for the traveler (to the traveler's company for JCAHO compliance purposes).

I believe that these regulations were created to assure quality of care that is provided to the hospitals that use travel nurses. I just don't like the fact that this may be at the expense of the smaller travel companies that provide the best customer service to the nurses.

Excellence in patient care should be the number one goal, and setting the same standards for healthcare agencies that the hospitals have to follow also may be just one more warranted step towards providing greater standards for all involved in the field of temporary staffing.

The Nursing Compact

In the year of 2000, Maryland, Texas, Utah and Wisconsin formed what is known now as the Nursing Compact. These four states were soon followed by many others to form a mutual recognition system. To date there are nineteen states that are in the Nursing Compact, with three others that have a bill signed by the governor, but which have not been put into effect. For a current list see the National Council of State Boards of Nursing's website at www.ncsbn.org.

For a traveling nurse, this is the best thing since the invention of the mobile phone! This means that as a resident of the state of Idaho, I can travel between nineteen different states without having to obtain a different license. This is only because my home residence is in a Compact state. If you live in Montana, which is not a Compact state, but have an Idaho license, it is *not* eligible for multi-state recognition. If you go to Texas and state that you are working under your "Idaho Compact License," you are actually practicing in Texas without a license, because your home is in Montana, instead of in Idaho.

If you have a multi-state license in one state and you move to another state in the Compact, your first license will no longer be valid. For instance, when I moved my residence from Arizona to Idaho, I received a letter from the State of Arizona, stating that my Arizona license had been inactivated due to the fact that I now have a multi-state license in Idaho. If your home state is a Compact state, your license will show "multi-state license," or something to that effect.

Your home state is the place where your house is or where you receive your mail if it's at a relative's house. Although the rules for home state aren't as strict as the tax home rules, I would still have ass much supporting information as possible to support your claim of a Compact state being your home state. This might include voter's registration, care registration, driver's license, and mail sent to your address.

Another confusing issue about the Nursing Compact is your state of original licensure. Your state of original licensure has *no* bearing on whether or not your license is a multi-state Compact license. In effect, if I moved my permanent residence to Montana, I would no longer be Compact eligible, even though my original license was granted in Idaho related to the fact that I'm no longer a resident of the state of Idaho.

The biggest safety advantage of the Nursing Compact is that nurses whose licenses have been revoked or suspended in one state will automatically have a record through a national database;

therefore making it more difficult for a nurse to get a new license in a different state after being convicted of a crime in another state or any other disciplinary action against their license.

When it comes to legal issues, although you practice under your Compact license, you are still required to practice until the rules of the state in which you are practicing in are effective. For example, although I have an Idaho Compact license, I am currently practicing in Tennessee. Therefore, at this time I would be held liable if I did *not* practice under the rules of the Tennessee State Board of Nursing, whereas Idaho State specific rules do not affect me at this time.

Be aware also that if you have a license in a non-Compact state that goes Compact, you will need to notify both boards as to which state is your home state. In other words, I also have an Oklahoma license where my parents live that is *not* Compact. When and if Oklahoma ever joins the Nursing Compact, I will need to notify both Idaho and Oklahoma that Idaho is my state of residence; otherwise I run the risk of my Idaho license being cancelled because I received my Oklahoma license a few years after my Idaho license. Some states will send you a request for your home state verification, but others will just cancel your oldest license. This has happened to some travelers who had to pay to get their legal home state licenses reinstated. It is imperative that you keep each state board of nursing informed of your permanent address at all times for this reason.

I have attempted to answer the basic questions about the Nursing Licensing Compact. If you have further questions, it is always best to call the state board. If you work in a state that is Compact and your license really is not a multi-state license, this will not only affect your license in that state, but *every* nursing license that you have. Ignorance is *not* bliss this time.

Performance Based Development System

This is a wonderful test that was developed by Dr. Dorothy del Bueno in an effort to test a nurse's critical thinking, interpersonal relation, and technical skills. The test consists of several short videos that are played, in which the nurse is required to recognize the problem, assess what interventions needed to take place, what he or she would expect the physician to order, prioritize how and when those interventions are to take place, while also taking into consideration conflict resolution, customer satisfaction, team building, and safety in performance and use of equipment.

The travel nurse will be required to take the test that most closely corresponds to that of their specialty. To date, testing is provided for adult Med/Surg, critical care, OR, OB, mental health, and ER. In the hospitals that I have researched, those whose specialty is pediatrics, rehab, or telemetry are required to take the Med/Surg test. Those whose specialty is step-down, surgical intensive care, medical intensive care, coronary intensive care, or neurological intensive care are all required to the critical care test.

Here is where the first problem lies: there is no test developed for every nursing field that there is. If I'm hired for telemetry and take the Med/Surg test, how does that prove my competency for the telemetry floor? If I'm hired for rehab and I take the Med/Surg test, how does that prove my competency for things such as how to manage the care of a patient who is trying to walk again versus a patient who is having an acute stroke? Some hospitals just give everyone the Med/Surg test as a "basic" nursing test, even though the nurse has been in the Psychiatric or OB field for ten years or so. Therefore, if they are going to use this for a competency-based assessment, they need to have it for the specialty that we say we are competent in and have been practicing in.

When you take this test, you will get about a twenty-second video of a patient who is having some kind of an acute distress, and you are supposed to figure out what is going on with that patient, what you should do first, and then progress from there until the patient is stable.

Here lays the second problem in the fact: that you are expected to write every little thing down that you can think of to do. You also have to think up of a diagnosis that you think the physician is going to assign to the patient. Remember, you have to do all this after viewing just once a short video, approximately 20 seconds' worth. Since when are nurses trained to diagnose what is wrong with the patient? Do you take notes or watch the video? I would think it is very difficult to accomplish both at the same time!

There is also a section which concentrates on prioritizing in "must do," "should do," or "could do." If a patient has a potassium level of 6.2 and another patient has a troponin level of 0.144 with a CKMB of 4.5, which is going to be my priority? Although the potassium level may cause some cardiac arrhythmias and would be considered a "should report," the elevated troponin and CKMB levels are more important and a "must report," related to the fact that they are indicative of a myocardial infarction.

These tests require you to write down not only what you would do in step-by-step format, but also why you are doing those things. One of the catches here is that you must write down all the little things. For example, for the an elevated potassium level you would not only notify the physician, who will probably order Kaexylate, but don't forget to also write down that you would hold the morning and evening doses of potassium.

To help study for this test, think about some of the situations that you have been in that require prioritization. What would you do or say if the charge nurse asked you to do orientation of a new nurse, but you have a really busy day and all of your patients have different procedures to go to on which you might have to accompany them? What would you say when a nurse comes up to you and asks you about another nurse, and what would you do if you witnessed a nurse yelling at a patient in the room?

Diseases that you might want to be familiar with and write out a care plan to study include heparin drips, insulin drips, diabetic coma, stroke, acute myocardial infarction, chest pain, increased intracranial pressure, digoxin toxicity, pneumothorax, congestive heart failure, chronic obstructive pulmonary disease, pulmonary embolism, renal failure, hemorrhage, pylonephritis, bladder retention, ilieus, thrombocytopenia, peritonitis, pain control, and sepsis.

What effect does this test have on travel nursing and why is it so controversial? It is because the test was designed to assess a nurse's strengths and weaknesses for an orientation process that is tailored to that nurse. But what the hospitals are now doing is using the test to "weed out" travel nurses that are "incompetent." This includes several nurses that have been "practicing incompetency" for twenty years. Excuse me? The state board of nursing says that I have been competent to practice nursing for twenty years, but a 20-second test says that I'm a danger to my patients?

I have heard numerous stories where the first week of orientation was going great, the hospital really liked the nurse, the nurse's professionalism and competence was being proofed daily with everyday situations, and then their contract was cancelled because all of a sudden some test says that they are incompetent. Now she has no job, but she still has a three-month lease on an apartment.

Let's just say that I have accepted a job in Naples, FL (several hospitals there are known for using the PBDS testing for travelers). To date, the average apartment lease is $1000/month plus a $200 deposit, and I will have to lease the apartment for 3 months in order to move in. This will be at a cost of $3200. After I lease the apartment, then I have to drive there from my home in Idaho. At the current rate of $0.48 for the 2600 miles, this would make my travel expenses $1248. At a rate of 500 miles per day, it will take me approximately 5.23 days to get from Idaho to Florida, which will mean 5 nights in motels at an average of $75/nightm for a total of $375. Then we will need to add $40/day for food, for a total of $200. That would mean my total for the trip and the three-month lease, not including rental furniture that will need to be returned, will be $5023.

My question now is, what nurse in her right mind would take a $5000 gamble on a test that is not being used as it was originally designed?

Unfortunately, there are some nurses who do take this gamble, and that is why the hospitals continue to use this testing system. I don't have a problem with a testing system to prove competency, but it needs to be arranged before a nurse drives across country only to have her contract cancelled. I don't even have a problem with the PBDS test, as long as it is being used to see where nurses are lacking and orientation is customized around what the nurses are lacking in. Travelers are expected to receive very minimal orientation and hit the floor running; therefore, extended customized orientation is not an option.

Chapter Sixteen

State Nursing Boards

Nursing Licensure Compact

One of the greatest things to have come along is the Nursing Licensure Compact. This is an agreement between states that gives you the right to move between certain states without having to obtain a new license. As simple as it may sound, there are a few things that you need to know about Compact states.

In the year of 2000, four states—Maryland, Texas, Wisconsin, and Utah—began a mutual recognition program. Since then, several other states have joined the Compact including Arizona, Arkansas, Colorado, Delaware, Idaho, Iowa, Kentucky, Maine, Mississippi, Nebraska, New Hampshire, New Mexico, North Carolina, North Dakota, Rhode Island, South Carolina, South Dakota, Tennessee and Virginia.

The main purpose of the Nursing Compact is to better regulate the movement of nurses through these states and to make it more difficult for an imposter to float through the different states. The main disadvantage for state boards is that the nurse doesn't have to get a new license; therefore, the income from licensing has decreased. However, I have noticed that a few years ago you could get a license in these areas for only $50.00 and now the licensing fees are $200 in several of the states.

For a nurse to have a multi-state license, that nurse has to reside in a Compact state. It is very important to nurses to understand that if you reside in a non-compact state, but have a license in a Compact state, that does *not* make your license a multi-state license. For example, if I reside in Oklahoma but have a Texas license, my license is good in Texas only because I do not reside in Texas; I'm only on assignment in Texas. In most states, your license will state "Multi-State License."

When you move from one Compact state to another Compact state, your "old" license will be good for 30 days. Within the first 30 days you must get a license in your new state. For instance, in 2005 I sold my house in Arizona and moved back to the house that I own in Idaho, thereby transferring my permanent residence from Lake Havasu City, AZ, to Pocatello, ID. I could practice in Idaho or any other Compact state for 30 days only before I had to get an Idaho license. If this is not done, then you can be convicted of practicing nursing without a license.

When you get to your assignment that is in a Compact state, you do not have to notify the state of your assignment, but you do need to do some research on the rules and regulations of that state. Right now I'm practicing in the state of Tennessee with my Compact license from Idaho. Although I'm not licensed in Tennessee, by practicing with my Idaho compact license I'm still responsible for following the rules and regulations of Tennessee.

To state that you reside in a Compact state isn't the same as having a tax home. Tax homes and residences can be the same, but also, you can be a resident of a state but be considered an itinerate worker because you are not duplicating expenses, which is required for a tax home. For you to claim a Compact state as your residence, you should have an address in a Compact state, driver's license, car registration, and voter's registration; the more information that you have to support your residence, the better. If you formerly resided in Arkansas and decided to go into travel nursing using your parents' address as your permanent address, chances are you vehicle registration, driver's license, and voter's registration are in Arkansas, because that is where you resided before hitting the road. If you do not pay your parents rent, you *cannot* claim that you have a tax home, but you can claim that that is your residence for the sake of having a Compact license.

If you have any questions on whether or not your license is Compact, do not hesitate to contact the board of nursing. You *cannot* be too careful when protecting your license!

State Board Information

State nursing board regulations vary from state to state. As a traveling nurse, it is your responsibility to find out what the laws are for the state in which you are interested in traveling to. To help you in this, I have listed here the states and their regulations as of October 2006.

State Nursing Boards

State Nursing Board Name

Alabama Board Of Nursing

Physical Address	**Mailing Address**
RSA Plaza, Ste. 250 770 Washington Ave. Montgomery, AL. 36104	P.O. Box 303900 Montgomery, AL 36130-3900
Work Phone	**Fax Number**
334-242-4060	334-242-4360
Website	**Original Verification**
www.abn.state.al.us	Yes

Fingerprint Card	**School Verification**	**CEUs Required**
No	Yes	Yes - 24hrs
Endorsement Amount	**License Time**	**Compact State**
$85.00	10 days	No
Picture	**All Licensed**	**Notary Signature**
No	Current Only	On copy of original license

State Nursing Board Name
Alaska Board Of Nursing

Physical Address
Robert B. Atwood Building
550 W. 7th Avenue, Suite 1500
Anchorage, AK 99501-3567

Mailing Address
550 W. 7th Avenue, Suite 1500
Anchorage, AK 99501-3567

Work Phone
907-269-8161

Fax Number
907-269-8197

Website
www.dced.state.ak.us

Original Verification
Yes

Fingerprint Card
Yes - two

School Verification
Yes

CEUs Required
Yes - 30

Endorsement Amount
$324.00

License Time
Walk Through

Compact State
No

Picture
Yes

All Licensed
Current Only

Notary Signature
Yes

State Nursing Board Name
Arizona Board Of Nursing

Physical Address
1651 East Morten Ave., Suite #150
Phoenix, AZ 85020

Mailing Address
1651 East Morten Ave., Suite #150
Phoenix, AZ 85020

Work Phone
602-331-8111

Fax Number
602-906-9365

Website
www.azbn.gov

Original Verification
Yes

Fingerprint Card
Yes

School Verification
No

CEUs Required
No

Endorsement Amount
$193.00

License Time
7 days

Compact State
Yes

Picture
No

All Licensed
Current Only

Notary Signature
No

State Nursing Board Name
Arkansas State Board Of Nursing

Physical Address
University Tower Building
1123 South University, Suite #800
Little Rock, AR 72204

Mailing Address
1123 South University, Suite #800
Little Rock, AR 72204

Work Phone
501-686-2700

Fax Number
501-686-2714

Website
www.arsbn.org

Original Verification
Yes

Fingerprint Card	**School Verification**	**CEUs Required**
Yes	No	Yes - 15hrs
Endorsement Amount	**License Time**	**Compact State**
$125	3 days	Yes
Picture	**All Licensed**	**Notary Signature**
Yes	Current Only	Yes

State Nursing Board Name
California Board Of Registered Nurses

Physical Address
1625 North Market Boulevard, Suite N-217
Sacramento, CA 94244-2100

Mailing Address
P.O. Box 944210
Sacramento, CA 95834-1924.

Work Phone
(916) 322-3350

Fax Number
(916) 574-8637

Website
www.rn.ca.gov

Original Verification
No

Fingerprint Card	**School Verification**	**CEUs Required**
Yes	Yes	30
Endorsement Amount	**License Time**	**Compact State**
$136	Walk through	
Picture	**All Licensed**	**Notary Signature**
Yes	Current Only	No

State Nursing Board Name
Colorado State Board Of Nursing

Physical Address	**Mailing Address**
1560 Broadway, Suite 880 Denver, Colorado	1560 Broadway, Suite 880 Denver, Colorado
Work Phone	**Fax Number**
303-894-2430	303-894-2821 (may fax applic.)
Website	**Original Verification**
www.dora.state.co.us	Yes

Fingerprint Card	**School Verification**	**CEUs Required**
No	No	No
Endorsement Amount	**License Time**	**Compact State**
$71.00	Walk through	Yes
Picture	**All Licensed**	**Notary Signature**
No	No	No

State Nursing Board Name
Conneticut Board of Examiners for Nursing

Physical Address	**Mailing Address**
410 Capitol Avenue, MS# 13PHO Hartford, CT 06134-0328	410 Capitol Avenue, MS# 13PHO Hartford, CT 06134-0328
Work Phone	**Fax Number**
(860) 509-7624	(860) 509-7553
Website	**Original Verification**
www.ct-clic.com	Yes

Fingerprint Card	**School Verification**	**CEUs Required**
No	Yes	No
Endorsement Amount	**License Time**	**Compact State**
$90.00	14 days	No
Picture	**All Licensed**	**Notary Signature**
Yes	Yes all states which you have been license in	No

State Nursing Board Name

Delaware State Board Of Nursing

Physical Address

861 Silver Lake Blvd
Cannon Building, Suite 203
Dover, DE 19904

Mailing Address

861 Silver Lake Blvd
Cannon Building, Suite 203
Dover, DE 19904

Work Phone

(302) 739-4522

Fax Number

(302) 739-2711

Website

Original Verification

Yes

Fingerprint Card

No

School Verification

No

CEUs Required

30 hrs

Endorsement Amount

$84.00

License Time

Walk Through

Compact State

No

Picture

No

All Licensed

Current Only

Notary Signature

Yes

State Nursing Board Name

District of Columbia

Physical Address

717 14th Street, NW, Suite 600
Washington, DC 20005

Mailing Address

717 14th Street, NW, Suite 600
Washington, DC 20005

Work Phone

(877) 672-2174

Fax Number

(202) 727-8471

Website

Original Verification

Yes

Fingerprint Card

No

School Verification

Yes

CEUs Required

24

Endorsement Amount

$176

License Time

Walk Through

Compact State

No

Picture

Yes

All Licensed

Only Current

Notary Signature

No

State Nursing Board Name
Florida State Board Of Nursing

Physical Address
4052 Bald Cypress Way, Bin C10
Tallahassee, Florida 32399-3260

Mailing Address
Post Office Box 6330
Tallahassee, Florida 32314-6330

Work Phone
(850) 245-4125

Fax Number
(850) 245-4172

Website
www.doh.state.fl.us

Original Verification
Yes

Fingerprint Card
Yes

School Verification
No

CEUs Required
Yes

Endorsement Amount
$212

License Time
30 days

Compact State

Picture
No

All Licensed
Current

Notary Signature
No

State Nursing Board Name
George State Board Of Nursing

Physical Address
237 Coliseum Drive
Macon, GA 31217-3858

Mailing Address
P.O. Box 13446
Macon, GA 31217-3858

Work Phone
(478) 207-1640

Fax Number
(478) 207-1660

Website
www.sos.state.ga.us

Original Verification
Yes

Fingerprint Card
No

School Verification
No

CEUs Required
No

Endorsement Amount
$60.00

License Time
14 days

Compact State
No

Picture
Yes

All Licensed
Only Current

Notary Signature
Yes

State Nursing Board Name
Hawaii Board Of Nursing

Physical Address
335 Merchant Street, Room 301
Honolulu, HI 96801

Mailing Address
PO Box 3469
Honolulu, HI 96801

Work Phone
(808) 586-3000

Fax Number
(808) 586-2689

Website
www.hawaii.gov

Original Verification
Yes

Fingerprint Card	**School Verification**	**CEUs Required**
No	No	None
Endorsement Amount	**License Time**	**Compact State**
$180.00	Walk Through	No
Picture	**All Licensed**	**Notary Signature**
No	Only original	No

State Nursing Board Name
Idaho State Board Of Nursing

Physical Address
280 North 8th Street, Suite 210
Boise, Idaho 83720

Mailing Address
PO Box 83720
Boise, Idaho 83720-0061

Work Phone
(208) 334-3110

Fax Number
(208) 334-3262

Website
www2.state.id.us/ibn

Original Verification
Yes

Fingerprint Card	**School Verification**	**CEUs Required**
Yes	Yes	No
Endorsement Amount	**License Time**	**Compact State**
$135	14 days	Yes
Picture	**All Licensed**	**Notary Signature**
Yes	Current Only	Yes

State Nursing Board Name

Illinois Department of Professional Regulation

Physical Address

James R. Thompson Center
100 West Randolph, Suite 9-300
Chicago, IL 60601

Mailing Address

James R. Thompson Center
100 West Randolph, Suite 9-300
Chicago, IL 60601

Work Phone

(312) 814-2715

Fax Number

(312) 814-3145

Website

www.idfpr.com

Original Verification

Yes

Fingerprint Card

Yes

School Verification

Yes

CEUs Required

None

Endorsement Amount

$64.00

License Time

14 days

Compact State

No

Picture

No

All Licensed

Only current for temporary

Notary Signature

No

State Nursing Board Name

Indiana State Board Of Nursing

Physical Address

Health Professions Bureau
402 W. Washington Street, Room W041
Indianapolis, IN 46204

Mailing Address

Health Professions Bureau
402 W. Washington Street, Room W041

Work Phone

(317) 232-2960

Fax Number

(317) 233-4236

Website

www.in.gov

Original Verification

Yes

Fingerprint Card

No

School Verification

No

CEUs Required

30hrs, including 8 in pharmacology

Endorsement Amount

$60.00

License Time

14 days

Compact State

Pending... Unknown implementation date

Picture

Yes

All Licensed

Only current

Notary Signature

For temporary license

State Nursing Board Name

Iowa Board Of Nursing

Physical Address

River Point Business Park
400 S.W. 8th Street, Suite B
Des Moines, IA 50309-4685

Mailing Address

River Point Business Park
400 S.W. 8th Street, Suite B
Des Moines, IA 50309-4685

Work Phone

(515) 281-3255

Fax Number

(515) 281-4825

Website

www.state.ia.us

Original Verification

Yes

Fingerprint Card

Yes
Report Class

School Verification

Yes

CEUs Required

45 hrs - Mandatory

Endorsement Amount

$169.00

License Time

5 days

Compact State

Yes

Picture

No

All Licensed

Only current

Notary Signature

No

State Nursing Board Name

Kansas State Board of Nursing

Physical Address

Landon State Office Bldg.
900 SW Jackson, Suite 551 S.
Topeka, KS 66612-1230

Mailing Address

Landon State Office Building
900 SW Jackson Street
Suite 1051

Work Phone

(785) 296-4929

Fax Number

(785) 296-3929

Website

www.ksbn.org

Original Verification

Yes

Fingerprint Card

No

School Verification

Yes

CEUs Required

30 hrs for renewal

Endorsement Amount

$75.00

License Time

Walk Through

Compact State

Yes

Picture

No

All Licensed

Only current for temp.

Notary Signature

Yes

State Nursing Board Name
Kentucky Board of Nursing

Physical Address
312 Whittington Parkway, Suite 300
Louisville, KY 40222

Mailing Address
312 Whittington Parkway, Suite 300
Louisville, KY 40222

Work Phone
(502) 329-7000

Fax Number
(502) 329-7011

Website
kbn.ky.gov

Original Verification
Yes

Fingerprint Card
Yes
(HIV/AIDS)

School Verification
Yes

CEUs Required
30hrs for renewal

Endorsement Amount
$175.00

License Time
14 days

Compact State
Yes

Picture
No

All Licensed
Only current for temp.

Notary Signature
No

State Nursing Board Name
Louisiana State Board of Nursing

Physical Address
5207 Essen Lane, Suite 6
Baton Rouge, LA 70809

Mailing Address
5207 Essen Lane, Suite 6
Baton Rouge, LA 70809

Work Phone
(504) 838-5332

Fax Number
(504) 838-5349

Website
www.lsbn.state.la.us

Original Verification
Yes

Fingerprint Card
Yes

School Verification
Yes

CEUs Required
5 to 15hrs

Endorsement Amount
$80.00

License Time
10 days

Compact State
No

Picture
No

All Licensed
Current Only

Notary Signature
Yes

State Nursing Board Name
Maine State Board of Nursing

Physical Address
158 State House Station
Augusta, ME 04333

Mailing Address
158 State House Station
Augusta, ME 04333

Work Phone
(207) 287-1133

Fax Number
(207) 287-1149

Website
www.state.me.us

Original Verification
Yes

Fingerprint Card
No

School Verification
Yes

CEUs Required
No

Endorsement Amount
$60.00

License Time
Walk through

Compact State
Yes

Picture
Yes

All Licensed
Only current

Notary Signature
Yes

State Nursing Board Name
Maryland State Board of Nursing

Physical Address
4140 Patterson Avenue
Baltimore, MD 21215

Mailing Address
4140 Patterson Avenue
Baltimore, MD 21215

Work Phone
(410) 585-1900

Fax Number
(410) 358-3530

Website
www.mbon.org

Original Verification
Yes

Fingerprint Card
No

School Verification
Yes

CEUs Required
None

Endorsement Amount
$100.00

License Time
Walk Through

Compact State
Yes

Picture
Yes

All Licensed
Only current

Notary Signature
No

State Nursing Board Name
Massachusets Nursing State Board

Physical Address
Commonwealth of Massachusetts
239 Causeway Street
Boston, MA 02114

Mailing Address
Commonwealth of Massachusetts
239 Causeway Street
Boston, MA 02114

Work Phone
(617) 973-0800

Fax Number
(617) 727-1630

Website
www.mass.gov

Original Verification
Yes

Fingerprint Card
No

School Verification
Yes

CEUs Required
15hrs for renewal

Endorsement Amount
$80.00

License Time
45 days

Compact State
No

Picture
No

All Licensed
Current Only

Notary Signature
No

State Nursing Board Name
Michigan CIS/Office of Health Services

Physical Address
Ottawa Towers North
611 W. Ottawa, 4th Floor
Lansing, MI 48933

Mailing Address
Ottawa Towers North
611 W. Ottawa, 4th Floor
Lansing, MI 48933

Work Phone
(517) 373-9102

Fax Number
(517) 373-2179

Website
www.michigan.gov

Original Verification
Yes

Fingerprint Card
No

School Verification
Yes

CEUs Required
25hr for renewal

Endorsement Amount
$48.00

License Time
21 days

Compact State
No

Picture
No

All Licensed
Yes - ALL

Notary Signature
No

State Nursing Board Name
Minnesota Board of Nursing

Physical Address
2829 University Avenue SE
Suite 500
Minneapolis, MN 55414

Mailing Address
2829 University Avenue SE
Suite 500
Minneapolis, MN 55414

Work Phone
(612) 617-2270

Fax Number
(612) 617-2190

Website
www.state.mn.us

Original Verification
Yes

Fingerprint Card
No

School Verification
Yes

CEUs Required
24hrs for renewal

Endorsement Amount
$100.00

License Time
7 days

Compact State
No

Picture
No

All Licensed
Current only

Notary Signature
No

State Nursing Board Name
Mississippi Board of Nursing

Physical Address
1935 Lakeland Drive, Suite B
Jackson, MS 39216-5014

Mailing Address
1935 Lakeland Drive, Suite B
Jackson, MS 39216-5014

Work Phone
(601) 987-4188

Fax Number
(601) 364-2352

Website
www.msbn.state.ms.us

Original Verification
Yes

Fingerprint Card
No (done at hospital)

School Verification
Yes

CEUs Required
None

Endorsement Amount
$125.00

License Time
5 days

Compact State
Yes

Picture
Yes

All Licensed
Current Only

Notary Signature
Yes

State Nursing Board Name
Missouri State Board of Nursing

Physical Address
3605 Missouri Blvd
P.O. Box 656
Jefferson City, MO 65102-0656

Mailing Address

Work Phone
(573) 751-0681

Fax Number
(573) 751-0075

Website
pr.mo.gov

Original Verification
Yes

Fingerprint Card
Yes

School Verification
Very some states

CEUs Required
None

Endorsement Amount
$67.00

License Time
Walk Through

Compact State
No

Picture
No

All Licensed
Copy of current for temp.

Notary Signature
Yes

State Nursing Board Name
Montana State Board of Nursing

Physical Address
301 South Park
Helena, MT 59620-0513

Mailing Address
P.O. Box 200513
Helena, MT 59620-0513

Work Phone
(406) 444-2071

Fax Number
(406) 841-2343

Website
www.nurse.mt.gov

Original Verification
Yes

Fingerprint Card
No

School Verification
Yes

CEUs Required
No

Endorsement Amount
$200

License Time
5 days

Compact State
No

Picture
Yes

All Licensed
All licenses in past 2 years

Notary Signature
Yes

State Nursing Board Name
Nebraska Health and Human Services System

Physical Address
Dept. of Regulation & Licensure, Nursing Section
301 Centenial Mall South

Mailing Address

Work Phone
(402) 471-4376

Fax Number
(402) 471-3577

Website
www.hhs.state.ne.us

Original Verification
Yes

Fingerprint Card
No

School Verification
Yes

CEUs Required
20hrs for renewal

Endorsement Amount
$76.00

License Time
Walk Through

Compact State
Yes

Picture
No

All Licensed
Notarized copy for temp.

Notary Signature
Yes

State Nursing Board Name
Nevada State Board of Nursing

Physical Address
2500 W. Sahara Ave., Suite 207
Las Vegas, NV 89102-4392

Mailing Address
2500 W. Sahara Ave., Suite 207
Las Vegas, NV 89102-4392

Work Phone
(702) 486-5800

Fax Number
(702) 486-5803

Website
nursingboard.state.n

Original Verification
Yes

Fingerprint Card
Yes

School Verification
Yes

CEUs Required
30hr for renewal

Endorsement Amount
$100.00

License Time
14 days

Compact State
Yes

Picture
No

All Licensed
Only current

Notary Signature
Yes

State Nursing Board Name
New Hampshire Board of Nursing

Physical Address
78 Regional Drive, BLDG B
Concord, NH 03302

Mailing Address
P.O. Box 3898
Concord, NH 03302

Work Phone
(603) 271-2323

Fax Number
(603) 271-6605

Website
state.nh.us/nursing

Original Verification
Yes

Fingerprint Card
Background check only

School Verification
No

CEUs Required
30hrs for renewal

Endorsement Amount
$155.00

License Time
7 days

Compact State
Yes

Picture
No

All Licensed
Only current

Notary Signature
No

State Nursing Board Name
New Jersey State Board of Nursing

Physical Address
124 Halsey Street, 6th Floor
Newark, NJ 07101

Mailing Address
P.O. Box 45010
Newark, NJ 07101

Work Phone
(973) 504-6586

Fax Number
(973) 648-3481

Website

Original Verification
Yes

Fingerprint Card
Background check only

School Verification
Yes

CEUs Required

Endorsement Amount
$195.00

License Time
45 days - No Temp.

Compact State
Pending

Picture
Yes

All Licensed
No

Notary Signature
Yes

State Nursing Board Name
New Mexico Board of Nursing

Physical Address
4206 Louisiana Boulevard, NE
Suite A
Albuquerque, NM 87109

Mailing Address

Work Phone
(505) 841-8340

Fax Number
(505) 841-8347

Website
www.bon.state.nm.us

Original Verification
Yes

Fingerprint Card
Yes

School Verification
Yes

CEUs Required
30hrs for renewal

Endorsement Amount
$141.00

License Time
14 days

Compact State
Yes

Picture
No

All Licensed
No

Notary Signature
No

State Nursing Board Name
New York State Board of Nursing

Physical Address
Education Bldg.
89 Washington Avenue
2nd Floor West Wing

Mailing Address
Education Bldg.
89 Washington Avenue
2nd Floor West Wing

Work Phone
(518) 474-3817 Ext. 120

Fax Number
(518) 474-3706

Website
www.op.nysed.gov

Original Verification
Yes

Fingerprint Card
No

School Verification
No

CEUs Required
6hrs - child abuse & infection control

Endorsement Amount
$135.00

License Time
60 days

Compact State
No

Picture
Yes

All Licensed
No

Notary Signature
Yes

State Nursing Board Name
North Carolina State Board of Nursing

Physical Address
3724 National Drive, Suite 201
Raleigh, NC 27612

Mailing Address
P.O. Box 2129
Raleigh, NC 27612

Work Phone
(919) 782-3211

Fax Number
(919) 781-9461

Website

Original Verification
Yes

Fingerprint Card
No

School Verification
Yes

CEUs Required
None

Endorsement Amount
$150.00

License Time
Walk through by appointment

Compact State
Yes

Picture
No

All Licensed
Yes

Notary Signature
No

State Nursing Board Name
North Dakota Board of Nursing

Physical Address
919 South 7th Street, Suite 504
Bismark, ND 58504

Mailing Address
919 South 7th Street, Suite 504
Bismark, ND 58504

Work Phone
(701) 328-9777

Fax Number
(701) 328-9785

Website
www.ndbon.org

Original Verification
Yes

Fingerprint Card
No

School Verification
Yes

CEUs Required
None

Endorsement Amount
$90.00

License Time
2 days

Compact State
Yes

Picture
No

All Licensed
None

Notary Signature
Yes

State Nursing Board Name
Ohio State Board Of Nursing

Physical Address
17 South High Street, Suite 400
Columbus, OH 43215-3413

Mailing Address
17 South High Street, Suite 400
Columbus, OH 43215-3413

Work Phone
(614) 466-3947

Fax Number
(614) 466-0388

Website
www.nursing.ohio.gov

Original Verification
Yes

Fingerprint Card	School Verification	CEUs Required
Yes	Yes	24hrs for renewal
Endorsement Amount	**License Time**	**Compact State**
$75.00	7-14 days	No
Picture	**All Licensed**	**Notary Signature**
Yes	Only current	Yes

State Nursing Board Name
Oklahoma State Board Of Nursing

Physical Address
2915 N Classen, Suite. 524
OKC, OK 73106

Mailing Address
2915 N Classen, Suite. 524
OKC, OK 73106

Work Phone
405.962.1800

Fax Number
405.962.1821

Website
www.ok.gov/nursing

Original Verification
Yes

Fingerprint Card	School Verification	CEUs Required
No	Yes	No
Endorsement Amount	**License Time**	**Compact State**
$95	14 days	No
Picture	**All Licensed**	**Notary Signature**
Yes	No	Yes

State Nursing Board Name
Oregon State Board of Nursing

Physical Address
800 NE Oregon Street, Box 25
Suite 465
Portland, OR 97232

Mailing Address
800 NE Oregon Street, Box 25
Suite 465
Portland, OR 97232

Work Phone
(503) 731-4745

Fax Number
(503) 731-4755

Website
www.oregon.gov/OSBN/

Original Verification
Yes

Fingerprint Card
Yes

School Verification
Yes

CEUs Required
None

Endorsement Amount
$135.00

License Time
10 days

Compact State
No

Picture
No

All Licensed
Current Only

Notary Signature
No

State Nursing Board Name
Pennsylvania State Board of Nursing

Physical Address
124 Pine Street
Harrisburg, PA 17101

Mailing Address
P.O. Box 2649
Harrisburg, PA 17101

Work Phone
(717) 783-7142

Fax Number
(717) 783-0822

Website
www.dos.state.pa.us

Original Verification
Yes

Fingerprint Card
No

School Verification
No

CEUs Required
None

Endorsement Amount
$35.00

License Time
14 days

Compact State
No

Picture
No

All Licensed
Current only

Notary Signature
No

State Nursing Board Name

Rhode Island Board of Nursing

Physical Address	**Mailing Address**
Registration and Nursing Education 105 Cannon Building 3 Capitol Hill	Room 105 3 Capitol Hill Providence, RI 02908
Work Phone	**Fax Number**
(401) 222-5700	(401) 222-3352
Website	**Original Verification**
www.health.ri.gov	Yes

Fingerprint Card	**School Verification**	**CEUs Required**
No	Yes	None
Endorsement Amount	**License Time**	**Compact State**
$93.75	14 days	Yyes
Picture	**All Licensed**	**Notary Signature**
Yes	All states licensed in.	Yes

State Nursing Board Name

South Carolina State Board of Nursing

Physical Address	**Mailing Address**
110 Centerview Drive Suite 202 Columbia, SC 29210	PO Box 12367 Columbia, SC 29210
Work Phone	**Fax Number**
(803) 896-4550	(803) 896-4525
Website	**Original Verification**
www.llr.state.sc.us	Yes

Fingerprint Card	**School Verification**	**CEUs Required**
No	Yes	No
Endorsement Amount	**License Time**	**Compact State**
$124.00	Walk through	Yes
Picture	**All Licensed**	**Notary Signature**
Yes	Only current for temp.	Yes

State Nursing Board Name
South Dakota Board of Nursing

Physical Address
4300 South Louise Ave., Suite C-1
Sioux Falls, SD 57106-3124

Mailing Address
4300 South Louise Ave., Suite C-1
Sioux Falls, SD 57106-3124

Work Phone
(605) 362-2760

Fax Number
(605) 362-2768

Website
www.state.sd.us/doh/

Original Verification
Yes

Fingerprint Card
Yes

School Verification
Yes

CEUs Required
None

Endorsement Amount
$125.00

License Time
Walk Through

Compact State
Yes

Picture
No

All Licensed
Only current

Notary Signature
No

State Nursing Board Name
Tennessee State Board of Nursing

Physical Address
426 Fifth Avenue North
1st Floor - Cordell Hull Building
Nashville, TN 37247

Mailing Address
426 Fifth Avenue North
1st Floor - Cordell Hull Building
Nashville, TN 37247

Work Phone
(615) 532-5166

Fax Number
(615) 741-7899

Website
www2.state.tn.us

Original Verification
Yes

Fingerprint Card
Yes

School Verification
Copy only required

CEUs Required
None

Endorsement Amount
$105.00

License Time
30 days

Compact State
Yes

Picture
Yes

All Licensed
Only current

Notary Signature
Yes

State Nursing Board Name

Texas Board of Nurse Examiners

Physical Address

333 Guadalupe, Suite 3-460
Austin, TX 78701

Mailing Address

333 Guadalupe, Suite 3-460
Austin, TX 78701

Work Phone

(512) 305-7400

Fax Number

(512) 305-7401

Website

texasonline.state.tx

Original Verification

Yes

Fingerprint Card

Yes

School Verification

Yes

CEUs Required

20hrs for renewal

Endorsement Amount

$200.00

License Time

14 days

Compact State

Yes

Picture

Yes

All Licensed

All appropriate licenses.

Notary Signature

Yes

State Nursing Board Name

Utah State Board Of Nursing

Physical Address

Heber M. Wells Bldg., 4th Floor
160 East 300 South
Salt Lake City, UT 84111

Mailing Address

Heber M. Wells Bldg., 4th Floor
160 East 300 South
Salt Lake City, UT 84111

Work Phone

(801) 530-6628

Fax Number

(801) 530-6511

Website

www.dopl.utah.gov

Original Verification

Yes

Fingerprint Card

Yes

School Verification

No

CEUs Required

15hrs for renewal

Endorsement Amount

$120.00

License Time

21 days

Compact State

Yes

Picture

No

All Licensed

Current Only

Notary Signature

No

State Nursing Board Name
Vermont State Board of Nursing

Physical Address
81 River Street
Montpelier, VT 05609-1106

Mailing Address
81 River Street, Drawer 9
Montpelier, VT 05609-1106

Work Phone
(802) 828-2396

Fax Number
(802) 828-2484

Website
vtprofessionals.org

Original Verification
Yes

Fingerprint Card
No

School Verification
No

CEUs Required
None

Endorsement Amount
$150.00

License Time
Walk through

Compact State
No

Picture
No

All Licensed
Copy of Current only

Notary Signature
No

State Nursing Board Name
Virginia Board of Nursing

Physical Address
6606 W. Broad Street, 4th Floor
Richmond, VA 23230

Mailing Address
6606 W. Broad Street, 4th Floor
Richmond, VA 23230

Work Phone
(804) 662-9909

Fax Number
(804) 662-9512

Website
www.dhp.state.va.us

Original Verification
Yes

Fingerprint Card
No

School Verification
No

CEUs Required
None

Endorsement Amount
$130.00
with other nursing license

License Time
No temp - can practice

Compact State
Yes

Picture
No

All Licensed
Copy of current only

Notary Signature
Yes

State Nursing Board Name

Washington State Nursing Commission

Physical Address	**Mailing Address**
Washington State Department of Health	Washington State Department of Health
Health Professions Quality Assurance	
310 Israel Rd.	Health Professions Quality Assurance

Work Phone	**Fax Number**
(360) 236-4740	(360) 236-4738

Website	**Original Verification**
fortress.wa.gov	Yes

Fingerprint Card	**School Verification**	**CEUs Required**
No	No	AIDs Education
Endorsement Amount	**License Time**	**Compact State**
$65.00	30 days	No
Picture	**All Licensed**	**Notary Signature**
Yes	Copy for temp.	No

State Nursing Board Name

West Virginia Board of Examiners for RNs

Physical Address	**Mailing Address**
101 Dee Drive	101 Dee Drive
Charleston, WV 25311	Charleston, WV 25311

Work Phone	**Fax Number**
(304) 558-3596	(304) 558-3666

Website	**Original Verification**
www.wvrnboard.com	Yes

Fingerprint Card	**School Verification**	**CEUs Required**
No	No	30hrs for renewal
Endorsement Amount	**License Time**	**Compact State**
$70.00	2 days	No
Picture	**All Licensed**	**Notary Signature**
Yes	Current notarized copy.	Yes

State Nursing Board Name
Wisconsin Department of Regulation and Licensing

Physical Address
1400 E. Washington Avenue
Madison, WI 53708

Mailing Address
P.O. Box 8935
Madison, WI 53708

Work Phone
(608) 266-0145

Fax Number
(608) 261-7083

Website
drl.wi.gov

Original Verification
Yes

Fingerprint Card
No

School Verification
No

CEUs Required
None

Endorsement Amount
$76.00

License Time
Walk through

Compact State
Yes

Picture
No

All Licensed
Copy of current.

Notary Signature
No

State Nursing Board Name
Wyoming State Board of Nursing

Physical Address
1810 Pioneer Ave
Cheyenne, WY 82002

Mailing Address
1810 Pioneer Ave
Cheyenne, WY 82002

Work Phone
(307) 777-7601

Fax Number
(307) 777-3519

Website
nursing.state.wy.us

Original Verification
Yes

Fingerprint Card
Yes

School Verification
Yes

CEUs Required
20hrs for renewal

Endorsement Amount
$190.00

License Time
7 days

Compact State
No

Picture
No

All Licensed
Notarized current only for temp

Notary Signature
Yes

Chapter Seventeen

On The Road Again With the Gang

Vernell From Alabama

Vernell is a psych nurse who has been traveling for a little over one year. She is with Supplemental Healthcare and doesn't plan on switching anytime soon. Her favorite city has been Raleigh, NC, with Baltimore, MD, being her least favorite.

She has traveled twice in her career, once in the late eighties, then again in early 2000. She worked for John Hopkins Hospital in Baltimore. The hospital was huge, but the people she worked with were very friendly and helpful. The residents and the staff were grateful for the help and welcomed her to the unit as a working member of the staff and not just as someone getting paid and wasting their time. Because it seemed to always be under construction, it was very difficult for her to get around in Baltimore. She was there for seven months and just beginning to understand how to get around when her time was up. One nurse and another nursing assistant took her under their wings and took her to sights of interest.

Her advice to a first timer includes, "Be careful; know your surroundings; don't be scared to explore and to realize nursing care is nursing care, just the surrounding and policies will be different."

Kimberly From Colorado

Kimberly is an orthopedic and spine nurse who states that money and location, followed by benefits and recruiter are most important to her. She has been traveling for almost five years, and prefers a one bedroom apartment that is paid for. Her favorite city has been Santa Barbara, CA, with Century City being her least favorite.

Her first travel assignment was a real eye-opener and she used all of her courage to find her survival resources. For a first timer, she states that it is important to jump in with both feet. Don't worry about the small stuff and use well-known travel friendly facilities, and by all means speak up if you are getting ditched on!

Lynn from Missouri

Lynn is a critical care nurse who rates money and location as priorities over benefits and a great recruiter. She has been traveling for almost five years with MedStaff, StarMed, Nursestat, RN Stat, and her current company, Health Specialists. Her disaster hospitals include Cox South, Springfield, MO; St. Louis University Hospital, St. Louis, MO; Raleigh Community Hospital, Raleigh, NC; Bothwell Regional Medical Center, Sedalia, MO; Golden Valley Hospital, Clinton, MO. Her favorite city has been Kansas City, with her least favorites being St. Louis, MO, and Raleigh, NC.

Her first travel experience was very stressful due to dangerous housing in the worst part of St. Louis, MO; the horrible drive of 1.5hrs to drive 17 miles from the apartment to the hospital; the traveling company which refused to move her, even though pimps, prostitutes, drug addicts hung around the door of the apartment building; the same company, which never paid her correctly so she spent long periods of time fighting with the payroll department trying to get the correct pay when she needed to be sleeping. Needless to say, she worked the thirteen weeks and went to another company. The company was StarMed. She liked the hospital through StarMed, but just didn't see eye-to-eye with the company.

What would she like to tell a first timer? "Be assertive. These companies and hospitals need you worse than you need them.

Remember, you are a valuable commodity. If RN's did not exist, none of these travel companies or hospitals could operate. Get along with the staff nurses you work with, but do not get sucked into their problems. My personal opinion now is that if a nurse works for a hospital that treats them badly and pays them poorly, they must be a masochist at heart. You will find very few places where the nurses are happy; if they were, you wouldn't be there as a travel nurse."

Cheryl from Louisiana

Cheryl is an RN who has been traveling for over two years. She prefers a one bedroom apartment for housing and places priorities on a great recruiter and pay scale. She is with Travel Nurse Solutions (previously World Health) and has absolutely no plans on changing. She previously worked with Professional Placement Resources, but has no plans on returning to them. The least friendly hospital that she has worked in was Kaiser Permanente in Oakland, CA, with her favorite being in Rancho Mirage, CA.

This is what she had to say about her first assignment: "I was a very new nurse, graduating in February 2001. I started my first travel assignment in early 2003 locally, just 30 miles from home. It was a very large teaching state hospital with primitive testing and limited orientation, but it was traveler friendly. The nurse patient ratio was 6-8 pts and she worked the night shift. On one of the busiest floors in the hospital, the tele floor, we handled a lot of new admissions and the hospital employed "admitting nurses," but only until 10-11pm, which was a major plus. They also were in nurse manager transition mode, which made it a little more challenging to get info and scheduling issues solved. I enjoyed it because it was fast-paced and challenging, to say the least. The location was top priority at that time, so money wasn't the biggest issue. However, being my first assignment, I found out quickly that travel companies make a chunk of change off of us and I learned real fast that the travel nurse industry is worth minding your p's and q's.

Advice to a first timer includes not being afraid of the unknown. Just jump in with both feet and give it your all. After all, you did it when you first started nursing school. Be *prepared* and keep in touch with other travel nurses with your same goals and make sure they are *positive* in thinking. Why? Positive produces positive and life has enough negatives already. Encouragement and support is much needed and sometimes the least provided. Enjoy life and your family! If you do, as a *person and* a nurse, what you don't get paid for, the rest takes care of itself. Go for it and don't look back! Tomorrow is a new day!

Judy from Florida

Judy is an ICU RN who prefers one bedroom paid-for housing. She placed money and benefits as being most important. Her disaster company is listed as Lifecare Associates. She is currently with RN Demand and does not plan to switch companies anytime soon.

Her least favorite hospital was Northern Arizona Medical Center, with King City, CA, being her least favorite city. Her favorite city has been Farmington, NM.

On her first travel assignment she was 1600 miles from home, knew no one, and was scared to death. She was afraid that she couldn't catch on in the short orientation, but managed just fine, which she survived because the hospital staff was very helpful and friend. She quickly learned and gained the confidence that *she could* do it!

What would she tell a first-timer? "Make sure everything you agree upon is relayed in your phone interview with the hospital and that it's in your contract. Make sure your hours are guaranteed in your contract. Listen to other travel nurses and learn from their mistakes."

Connie from Nebraska

Connie is an OR nurse who has been traveling for almost a year. She takes the housing stipend and travels in her RV. She currently travels with RN Demand and her favorite city has been Sandpoint, Idaho.

She had a one-day orientation with three staff nurses on her first assignment, and none were much good at teaching nor had a complete working knowledge of the unit. It took about two weeks to put it all together, then things started going great and she extended her assignment. The trick to surviving an assignment, according to Connie, is to keep smiling and realize that not every day is going to be your best day. And most importantly, ask questions, ask questions, and then ask more questions.

GG from North Carolina

GG is a Stepdown/Telemetry nurse who prefers to be housed in a two bedroom apartment, which the company provides. She has been traveling for almost two years, and places money and location above benefits and a great recruiter. She is now traveling with Cross Country TravCorp, but is open to other companies. Her favorite city has been High Point, NC, with Cape Fear Valley and Fayetteville, NC, being her least favorite.

Her first travel nursing experience was fun, exciting, and nerve-racking, but a great learning experience. Her advice to new travelers is to always check on your floating status and to what unit you are assigned. Some hospitals will put your license in jeopardy. When you are orienting to the unit, make sure that you know *where all* the policies, procedure, and protocol books are located at a moments notice.

Tekoa from Tennessee

Tekoa is an NICU nurse who has been traveling for over two years. She is now with Strategic Healthcare after leaving the disaster of American Mobile. Her favorite cities have been Washington, DC, and San Francisco, CA, with her least favorite being Corpus Christi, TX.

Her first assignment was fun, exciting, and completely underpaid, but a great learning experience. She would like to remind all first timers to talk to as many people as possible and *read* your contract before signing it.

Judy from Florida

Judy is an OB nurse with over a year's worth of experience. She travels in an RV and placed location and money as priorities over a great recruiter and benefits. Her worst hospital was Naples Community. Her favorite city was San Diego, CA, and named Crossville, TN as her least favorite.

She traveled from South Florida to California in an RV with her husband and dog for her first assignment. It was very exciting to see new country while they traveled and settled in to a campground and located the hospital. The first day was a little scary, but it was also exciting to meet new people, see how things worked there, and say "she am a travel nurse." They saw many places that they had only read, seen or heard about in the year they were in California. They made many wonderful memories together. The work experience has made her see and do some things differently, and take those to new places and share with others. She loves the flexibility and adventures travel nursing gives to her.

Kathy from Idaho

Kathy is a telemetry nurse who prefers a one bedroom apartment. She has been traveling for two years and is now with National Healthcare but is looking to switch. She states that has been unhappy with both Medical Express and National Healthcare. She places money and benefits over location and a great recruiter. Her favorite city has been Seattle, WA, with Santa Clara, CA and Kaiser being her least favorite city/assignment.

Her first assignment at Oschner Clinic Foundation in New Orleans, just five months after Katrina, was great. It was the most wonderful place to work. She would like to remind all new traveling nurses to get a signed contract *before* you leave for the assignment.

Twana from Illinois

Tawan is a labor and delivery nurse who has been traveling for less than a year with Trustaff and is looking for a new company.

She places location as most important, with money and benefits coming in next. Her favorite city has been Lake Jackson, TX.

Her first assignment was a very new experience. She had to deal with the darker elements of Trustaff. Everything that that company provided came out of her wages, and they only have the tax advantage as an option. She found herself looking at what seemed to be a very small paycheck. She changed recruiters and dealt with a different housing person and managed to survive because she was working in a great hospital. The nurses at Lake Jackson were very traveler-friendly, as well as the management. "If you're looking for a great small town feeling, this is the place!"

What would she like to tell a first timer? "Have everything in writing. You must make sure that sure that your recruiter answers all of your questions to your satisfaction. Don't fall for the sales pitch. Take care of yourself because the company will not at all times."

***Note from Epstein: As stated before in this book, hospitals pay the company a bill rate; all benefits, company expenses, and your wages come out of that bill rate. Twana is correct in that you need to keep the company honest! If you truly think that your pay rate is low, go to www.pantravelers.org and use their salary calculation tool and see if the bill rate sounds right. California bill rates now are at about $70 and Florida bill rates are about $50. Everything else is USUALLY in between.*

Leslie from Pennsylvania

Leslie is a progressive care unit nurse who places location and a great recruiter as priorities. She has been traveling for under a year with American Mobile and stays in a two bedroom apartment. Her favorite city has been Beaufort, SC.

Her first traveling experience was a very positive one in that she found a job within a week of looking. Her recruiter was wonderful and talked to her until she was ready to go. The hospital was filled with traveling nurses and she had a great time. She would like to remind all nurses to make sure that everything you want is in your contract.

Dawn from Wisconsin

Dawn is a dialysis nurse who placed location and recruiter has most important, with money and benefits secondary. She has been traveling for a year and a suite is fine. She has been traveling with Foundation Medical Staffing, but would consider another travel company. Her favorite place has been Anchorage, AK, with Madison, WI, being her least favorite.

Her first travel experience was totally awesome. She appreciated many of the people she met there, both at work and at play. Most seemed "nicer" there than in other places. She learned to cross-country ski, caught her first salmon, fell into the water and learned to dip net. She saw her first moose and their babies! The summers are fantastic in Alaska!

She thinks that it's a plus for a traveler to have a personality that works well either alone or with others, as we never know what's going to happen on assignment. Also, being outgoing is helpful so you can initiate conversation, as well as participate in outside activities.

Mia from Ohio

Mia is a progressive care and intensive care nurse who travels mostly for the money. Instead of company- supplied housing, she takes the housing stipend and finds her own. She has been traveling for almost five years with American Mobile, but is open to traveling with another company. Her favorite assignment was in Raleigh, NC, with Naples Community Hospital in Naples, FL listed as her worst.

Naples Community Hospital is an absolute nightmare! The director on her floor was completely rude, unwilling to work with staff etc... The nurses-to-patient ratios are out of control. They make you take a very hard written out test which is pass or fail...and if you fail, they cancel your contract on the spot! It was the worst travel assignment ever.

For first timers, she would just like to remind them the *get everything* in writing!

Connie from Mississippi

Connie is an OR, PACU, and Endo nurse who places money and benefits as top priority. She takes the housing stipend and uses her RV. She has been traveling for almost a year and is not dedicated to any one travel company. Her favorite city has been Birmingham, AL.

About her first assignment she states, "My first assignment was in Montgomery, AL, at Jackson Hospital. They were very busy and very disorganized. The staff was friendly and worked very hard and they worked well as a team. The surgeons were arrogant and the reason she did not re-sign on. There are too many other places to work to put up with that type of treatment. Birmingham and St. Vincent East was great! There were a lot of great team players. The surgeons were mostly very nice and competent. I enjoyed working there. i was treated fairly like one of them. They taught me so much. The only bad thing was that I had a 30-minute commute to work because I was staying in my RV and that was the nearest park."

She would like to remind first-time travelers to stay focused and work hard. "Do not take your work home with you, and have fun!"

Kayci from New York

Kayci works in the Emergency Room and has been traveling for over two years. She takes the housing stipend and finds her own apartment. She travels with American Mobile now, after her bad experience with Cirrus Medical Staffing. Her favorite city has been Charlotte, NC.

Her first travel nursing experience was great fun. She was so happy that she had taken the risk and did it. Taking that first assignment is half the battle. Her first job was in NYC and it was *great*. She loved her recruiter, loved her apartment, and loved the hospital.

What would she tell a first timer? "*Please, please*...if you would like to re-sign at a certain hospital, *be flexible!* That is one reason why hospitals hire travelers. The more flexible you are the more money they are willing to offer you and better scheduling. Be a team player...and *work hard* and everything will run smoothly!"

Tasha from North Carolina

Tasha is a cardiac step-down and telemetry nurse who places importance on money and a great recruiter over benefits and location. She takes the one bedroom housing that is supplied to her by Nurse Choice. During her almost 2 years of traveling, Phoenix, Arizona has been her favorite assignment, with Dover, Delaware being her least favorite.

She took an assignment back in her home state of Delaware so the transition would be a little more smooth, being that she was in a familiar place trying something new. The hospital, Beebe Medical Center, was very traveler-friendly and the orientation was excellent, so her first experience wasn't too hectic. The staff was very welcoming and friendly, and it probably helped that the hospital is near the beach. Many of the other nurses on her floor were travelers also and a handful were repeat travelers to that facility. She chose to begin her travel experience with American Mobile Healthcare, which is a pretty good company, but she never really felt a connection with her Recruiter and she probably talked to her assistant more than she spoke with her.

She would like to emphasize that new travelers should do their research before signing with any company or facility and to make sure to find a recruiter with whom you mesh and who is out for your best interest.

Tricia from New York

Tricia is a CVICU nurse who has been traveling for under a year. She places priorities on location and money over benefits and a great recruiter. She has been with Cross Country Trav Corp and has no intention of switching. Her favorite city has been Baltimore, MD.

Her first travel assignment was in New York at New York Presbyterian-Columbia. It was an absolutely great hospital. For Tricia, leaving was very hard related to the fact that it was very traveler friendly. She worked in the PACU with a great staff and she absolutely loved it.

She would like to remind first time travelers to do their research on the companies that they plan to sign up with and the hospital that you want to work at and *read your contract.* If it is not what was agreed on, *do not sign it!* And most importantly, enjoy the world of travel nursing.

Eva from Tennessee

Eva is an Emergency Room nurse who places her priorities as money and benefits secondary to location and a great recruiter. She has been traveling for one year and takes the one bedroom paid for apartment. Her favorite hospital was in Hartford, Connecticut, with her least favorite being Sacramento, California. Although she loved the town of Sacramento, she wasn't too fond of the hospital.

Her first travel assignment was an awesome experience in New Britain, CT. She had to move after two weeks to a better location, but that was okay. New Britain General Hospital (now the hospital of Central Connecticut) was extremely traveler-friendly. The staff and the doctors were wonderful, friendly, and warm. Her second assignment was at Mercy General in Sacramento, CA, and it was her first non-traveler friendly hospital. There were four to six doctors that she worked with that were very nasty to all nurses.

She would like to tell all first time travelers to gather a notebook together with sections. Keep all your license, shot records, TB, resume, etc. in there; you will need it a lot! It makes it very handy to be organized.

Sigurid from Nebraska

Sirgurid is a step-down, telemetry, and med/surg nurse who has been traveling for under a year. She takes the one bedroom paid-for apartment and places location as top priority. She is currently with Trustaff.

Unfortunately, her first travel assignment was "Nightmare At Valley View." They had just received their JCAHO certification, but she isn't sure how they got it. The med/surg/telemetry unit was a disaster as it was understaffed, unorgranized, with a very high acuity. To top it all off, the nursing staff was very unfriendly, not helpful, and travel nurses were treated with absolutely no respect. What even made it worse was the fact that when there was a discrepancy on the Kronas, her recruiter and travel company didn't back her up, even with the signed time sheets for all the overtime. She was then terminated by the hospital for speaking to HR about her frustrations. The travel company used her last pay check to cover the last two weeks of the housing contract and left her with no money, and then they found her a new job within a week which did not require her to move, which did help out things.

Things she would like to tell a first time traveler include:

1. Get it in writing and do not believe that your agency will back you up when it comes to an issue that might mean the hospital will terminate their contract with the agency, not just with you. Make sure you have everything done and are ready to go with several companies before you take your first assignment, meaning physical, immunizations, respirator fit testing, and all the application and skill testing done so you can be ready to go with any of your chosen companies at a moments notice.
2. Research the web sites by travel nurses for travel nurses, such as this www.highwayhypodermics.com, ultimatenurse.com, nurseforum.com, Delphi etc. It pays to heed the advice of seasoned travelers who can tell you what companies are good, what hospitals to stay away from.
3. Have realistic expectations. Know that if the pay and bonuses are high there are more than likely issues for travelers and staff alike and that staff may have attitude toward travel nurses in general, so stick with your fellow travel nurses, bond, share, complain to one another, but do not voice your opinion in front of staff as they will tattle on you to management and among themselves, which can make your life a living hell there.
4. Make sure that you have in writing that the facility must call you to discuss schedule changes and that you have the right to refuse changes. A traveler must be flexible, but one does not have to be inconvenienced by changes made by management without permission. Such changes mean you have no life, you cannot make plans to explore, and you might end up with a long stretch of shifts without a day off. Get in

writing how many shifts you will work in a row (two on, two off, etc.). For example, I do not like working 4 nights in a row with a 48-hours guaranteed contract. It is too fast paced and my body does not do well with 4 twelve's in a row. Know your limits and stick to them.

5. Make sure you know just what your company's policy is on contracts being cancelled early or without just cause. Save at least $1000 dollars, just in case, for relocation expenses to cover any expenses not covered by your company. Sirgurid stated, "In my case, I still had six shifts to work or two weeks before my contract was up, so the company used my paycheck to pay the last two weeks of my housing and the cat deposit, which was supposed to be taken out over the 8 weeks of the contract but had not been, so I lost the entire paycheck which I had already written checks for bills and mailed. Overdrafts cost me more money."

6. Find out what the state you are working in allows for per diem on the tax advantage system and make you company do it right.

7. Utilize the Tax Advantage System if you reside in another state as your primary residence. Learn about it. Ask a seasoned traveler how it works if your recruiter does not explain it well. Sometimes they encourage it when it saves them money but is not to your advantage, so always check out what is best for your situation—not theirs.

8. Things you will definitely need to bring: digital camera, lap top computer, make sure local phone is in your contract unless you have a cell plan that does not have roaming charges. Always ask about what is included in furnished apt., i.e. dishes plates, etc. Sirgurid also stated, "In my case, I elected to take my pots and pans, dishes, and silverware, coffee pot, and cooking utensils, a cookie sheet etc. as it saved me $160 a month on my housing. What size bed and if linens are included. It all depends on if you drive to your assignment or fly. If flying, make sure your travel company has a rental car waiting for you when you arrive and understand what it will cost you to drive it."

9. My two requests: A washer/dryer in the apt. unit and high speed internet. I am willing to pay a little more to not have to go to a laundromat or a community apt. laundry facility. Basic cable should be included, as well as utilities and local phone when possible. In some remote areas you may have to use Wi-Fi for internet, so check out what is available, and in some areas cell phones drop call no cell towers.
10. Remember the agency you work for is out to make money too, so if it is not in writing they may renege on admitting they ever said it or promised it to you.

Jennifer from Maryland

Jennifer is an NICU nurse with almost two years of experience who places her priorities on money and a great recruiter. Although she was once with American Mobile, she currently travels with On Assignment. Her favorite places have been Palm Springs, CA, and Long Beach, CA, with her least favorite being Santa Barbara, CA.

Her first assignment was horrendous! The housing was far from the facility and traffic was even worse. She was tired by the time she got to work. That assignment lasted only two weeks. That was it, she couldn't take it any longer. That was her very first travel assignment, almost 10 years ago. Since then she's learned the ropes and she says she is still learning!

She would like to remind the first time traveler to get everything *in writing!* Be sure to do the interview with the facility so you can have all of your questions answered. Absolutely do not take the assignment if you have any doubts!

David from Minnesota

David is a Critical/Intensive Care nurse who has been traveling for almost two years. He places his priorities on a great salary and recruiter. He is fine with a suite from Medical Express. His favorite city has been Denver, CO, with his least favorite being New Bedford, MA.

His fist assignment ended up with him in a very unsafe city and a hospital with very poor management and poor patient care.

His first introduction to the city involved a car of gang-bangers holding a knife out their car window, and him unsure how to get out of his contract. Thank goodness that the city was surrounded by great things to visit.

David would like to remind travelers to be very well prepared as a nurse first and foremost!

Cynthia from Pennsylvania

Cynthia is an ER nurse who has been traveling for less than a year. Most important to her travels are a great recruiter and location, followed by salary and benefits. She prefers a two bedroom apartment. She is not currently traveling because of her first travel experience. She doesn't have a favorite hospital, but did not do well in Baltimore, MD or Reading, PA.

After her first travel assignment she came up with her own not-so-short questionnaire. Her first experience cost her time, gasoline, mileage on her car, and worst of all, her own self-worth as an RN. She was a small hospital ER nurse (5 bed ER in a 25 bed hospital), and her first assignments were in two metropolitan ERs and one was even a trauma center! She was cancelled by the two hospitals and put on a year probation, with the requirement of two references in order to get back with the same agency. The agency paid well, but the nurse had to be able to function "competently" on the first day. For future reference, from now on she figures that she has to walk on water and turn water it into wine or she will not—repeat, will not travel again. She would sooner starve on the unemployment line than have a horrible experience like this again.

What did she learn from her first experience? Beware of those bearing too-good-to-be-true promises and verify *everything*. She also suggests making a very large list of questions to be answered by recruiters.

***Note From Epstein: I included this for one very important reason. I'm not sure how much experience Cynthia had as a nurse, but it is so important to be confident with your skills and to have at least one year of med/surg, rehab, psych experience if* *that is your specialty of TWO years of the more critical care fields, including ICU, PICU, ER, OB/GYN, and OR. As a traveling nurse, you are expected to hit the floor running and know what you are doing. Cynthia I'm sure is a great nurse who just got in a little over her head and couldn't tread water fast enough without a support system. I'm sure that she would have done fine in a small ER like she was from, but the mistake that she and the company she worked for made was putting her in too deep of water for her first assignment. YOU have to be realistic about how much you really can handle as a nurse and don't let the recruiters SELL you to the highest bidder and biggest hospital because that is what they have available. There are plenty of other agencies who have a lot of other assignments available.*

David from Texas

David is an ER and ICU nurse who places salary, location, and a great recruiter as his priorities. He prefers to travel in his RV and take the housing stipend. He has been traveling for six years. He has traveled with several companies and really isn't loyal to any one. His favorite cities having included Reno, NV, Redding, CA, Long Beach, CA, Paris, TX, and Lancaster, CA, with his least favorite being Oakland, CA and Rutland, VT.

His first travel job was in Providence, RI in 2001. It's a good thing that he was not scared off that easily. He was sent there on a four week assignment and essentially felt as though he was dumped out to fend for myself. He had a recruiter that never returned calls and he was a good ol' southern boy cast into a world of people. He had no idea what they were like. But, due to his will to make it in the travel world and his expertise of the job, he hung in there and made the best out of a bad situation. David made loads of new friends and saw some of the most beautiful places that he had no idea existed. Only meeting new friends and seeing great places kept him hoping to fine tune this travel business. Today, six years later, he knows that taking the plunge to start traveling was the best nursing career move he ever made.

What would he tell a first timer? "Yes, I know the security you feel you have in that everyday job as a staff member! Been there done that. Fear enters your mind with the thought of the unsure or the unknown, but once you get the nerve and get past that to set forth the spirit to venture into the world and get your feet wet on new experiences, you will see nursing in a whole new light. Wherever I go, it's the travelers that are smiling. Not just because of the money, but more for the freedom they have over the regular staff nurse that is bound to that administration, or that mandatory meeting, or that mandatory overtime, or that short staffed unit. Wherever I go, I am usually able to relay my stories to some of the staff nurses, and sometimes I get calls from them that they have taken up the road also."

Connie from Mississippi

Connie is a MS, PACU, Endo. nurse who places her priorities on a great salary and benefits. She takes the housing stipend and travels in her RV. She has been traveling under a year with Travel Nurse Solutions.

She absolutely loved her first travel assignment and meeting new people and learning different ways to do things. Change is always good! That is why she believes that travelers should never re-sign with a hospital. Do your thirteen weeks and move on. It is a great way to improve your resumé. Do not let employees (staff) hurt your feelings about being a traveler. Remember, they would probably love to be able to do the same. She encourages them to take the plunge one day. Just keep in the front of your mind, no matter how bad things go, that contracts only last thirteen weeks!

Lauren from Texas

Lauren is an ER nurse whose number one priority in a travel company is benefits. She takes the standard one bedroom housing that Cross Country Trav. Corp provides. She has been with American Mobile, but wouldn't go back. Her favorite assignment was Hartford Children's Hospital, with her least favorite being anything in Texas.

Her first travel experience at Cambridge, MA was horrible. There were not enough nurses, and they really were rude. She felt like her license was in jeopardy several times. The hospital was old, like a cave, dirty, and dark.

She would like to remind newbies not to get involved with the staff on management issues. Trust no one until you are sure. Do your work, keep your head down and smile! Fake it until you make it!

Veronica from Arkansas

Veronica is an ICU nurse who places location and a great recruiter as most important to her. She takes the two bedroom housing and doesn't mind paying some for the extra room. She has been traveling for over ten years and is currently with PPR (Professional Placement Resources). She previously worked with RN Network and Medstaff, which she will not return to. Although her experience with the hospital was not very pleasant at the Univ. of Calif. San Francisco (UCSF), she loved being in the city of San Francisco. She also prefers not to travel to the southern part of the United States.

Her first assignment was with RN Network, and she feels like they did a "bait and switch" on her. She had turned down Walnut Creek, CA and left for an "assignment" in San Francisco. She packed, rented out her house, and hit the road. Upon arrival they stated, "Oops, we got the wrong hospital!" She feels like they were going to leave her stranded in California unless she took the Walnut Creek job, which she did agree to take. When she finally got the UCSF through Med Staff, they mailed her checks thousands of mile away to her home instead of where she was, causing severe financial problems, and then they left her "homeless" when UCSF cancelled the contract due to a lack of funds and a rash of funds and a rash of hiring new grads. She was told by Med Staff that she had twenty-four hours to get out or they would hold her paycheck.

What would she tell a first timer? "Never travel with RN Network or Med Staff. Sign up with 2 agencies and be ready to go with both if something happens. The other can pick you up and even assume the apartment you are in! Remember, high rates of pay or big bonuses are because the hospital is bad and cannot attract nurses. Good hospitals don't have to pay as much and will take time to get into. This is why UCSF has dozens of openings and St. Francis has only one or two in any given time."

***Note From Epstein: I have not talked to Veronica, but her story is just a reminder to READ YOUR CONTRACT. Make sure you know where you are going and with whom your contract is. Contracts are contracts, and if the agency put in the wrong hospital they would still need to pay for your travel expenses to the assignment and pay for that contract until they could find something agreeable to you. I would then seriously consider whether or not you want to continue to travel with that company. To me, it would depend if it's a one time thing or something that has happened to you before.*

Ritchie the Nomad

Ritchie is an ER nurse who places his priorities on salary and a great recruiter. He classifies himself as a "Mountain West Nomad" as he travels around in his RV. He doesn't have a company that he really prefers, but knows that he will never return to American Mobile. His favorite assignment was in Stanford, CA, with his least favorite in Reno, NV.

His first assignment was for a great small hometown agency with great pay and excellent housing in a little old cow town in Wyoming. He would like to remind new travelers that even experienced travelers get shafted by recruiters who are so sweet and can lie and smile and stab and get you to let your guard down. "This is a business arrangement. The recruiter and facility is *not* your friend, even though it may seem that away. Dang, I should have learned that myself!" he states. He was recently drowning when a recruiter was smiling as she threw him a concrete life ring.

Colleen from New York

Colleen is a med-surg nurse who has been traveling for under a year with O'Grady Peyton. Her priorities include salary and location. Her favorite place has been Baltimore, MD.

She has learned a lot about herself as a nurse that she didn't see before she started traveling. She learned to be flexible, assertive, independent, and her assessment skills improved. She knew that she was a good nurse, but being a traveler is different and you learn that you are stronger than you may have originally thought. She states, "Don't be scared; just go for it!"

Sue from Connecticut

Sue is a med/surg nurse who places her priorities on location and salary. She takes the one bedroom housing paid for by Med Staff. Her favorite place has been San Francisco, CA, with Alta Bates, CA, and Bakersfield, CA, being her least favorite.

Her first assignment was crazy and overwhelming. She and her friend were so excited to have their first assignment at Memorial Sloan Kettering in NYC, then they had nine to twelve cancer patients who were very sick. To make things worse, there were no respiratory therapists and the IV pumps were only for the patients who were receiving chemotherapy. The unit had close to 40 rooms, but only one med room. She had to run back and forth constantly, and to make things worse, the unit had only one Glucometer. The charge nurse could not stand them and made them feel stupid. Being travelers, they always got the admissions. It was all paper charting, and tons of it. The nursing assistants were lifesavers. It was great that she traveled with her friend. They almost had the exact same schedule on the same unit and were there to help each other when they could. When times got bad, they were always there for each other.

What would she tell a first timer? "Do not complain about floating. Be flexible and act like you don't care. Managers and other staff members do not like complainers. Be prepared to float; it comes with traveling. Sometimes floating is a relief if you work on a crazy unit. Hospitals know they cannot float you to an area where you have no experience; your assignment must be modified in this case. Ask a million questions during the hospital interview and write everything down. Don't feel that you have to accept an offer just because you interviewed; don't let your recruiter pressure you. Don't trust the company or your recruiter. The company wants to make money, as well as your recruiter. In most cases your recruiter is a salesperson, not your friend. Beware of hospitals that offer high pay rates...there is a reason. Listen to other travelers. If they have had a horrible experience, most likely you will too. Many staff nurses do not like travelers. They are jealous. Just ignore them and don't let their attitude bother you. Try to get on the good side of the unit manager. It will pay off (great reference, great schedule). Follow all unit/hospital procedures and look them up if you are not sure. Do not follow your old hospital's policies/procedures; this can get you in trouble. Explore the city/town you are in and have fun!"

Cheryl from Kansas

Cheryl is a labor and delivery nurse who places priorities on a great location and salary. She has been traveling with Aureus Medical for almost five years. Her favorite city has been Cortez, CO, with her least favorite being Springfield, MO.

Her first assignment was a little rough in that she didn't get much orientation and she worked by herself at nights. Thank goodness the physicians were friendly and helped her find things. The staff was friendly and supportive, but the drive back to KS was a killer. She would like to remind nurses to specify what you want as far as job limitation on your contract. Everything must be in writing.

Kathy from Wisconsin

Kathy is a neuro/med/surg nurse who places her priorities on benefits and location. She takes the one bedroom paid-for housing provided by Emerald Heath Services. She didn't have quite as good a luck with RTG Medical and Bestaff. Her favorite hospital has been San Rafael, CA, with Chico, CA, being her least favorite.

Her first travel assignment was rough as she felt like her recruiter lied to her and left her stranded three hours from home in a hospital that was the worst she has ever been in. She would like to remind all new nurses to get everything in writing, and even then the travel company can still lie to you. Beststaff's contract stipulated an eighth-week contract of twelve hour nights. When she arrived at Novato she was working days, Pms, Nocs and eight and twelve hour rotating shifts. Then she found out that

Beststaff had typed the wrong ending date on the contract with the hospital so she was left without work for two weeks. Beststaff pretended to be a small southern company that had Christian values, but to her they were they just the opposite. They lied about everything, including the apartment, which was a dive and they wouldn't do anything about it when she brought that to their attention. The doors didn't lock, the balcony was rotting wood, the carpet and flooring had sharp tacks sticking up and you couldn't go barefoot, etc.

Michelle from Nevada

Michelle is an NICU nurse who counts salary and a great recruiter has her top picks. She takes the two bedroom housing from Aureus Medical. Her favorite city has been Las Vegas.

Her first assignment was in Seattle, WA at Evergreen Hospital with HRN. First of all, she had a great recruiter, Summer, who is regrettably no longer with them. She was very on-the-ball, helped her figure out the ropes, and got her the greatest little apartment in a fabulous neighborhood. She went to work with the night crew, had awesome co-workers and stayed on for a total of six months. It was a great first time experience. She was so glad it wasn't a horror story like some nurses have!

She would like to remind first timers not to ever go into a facility and tell the staff repeatedly, "Well, back at (blank facility) we did it this way." Staff hates to hear that, even if it is true. It just grates on the nerves. She had a traveler at her old hospital once who always said, with her thick Bronx accent, "Well, back in New York..." (you fill in the blank). Everything was done differently there, apparently. If you have to absolutely add your two-cents about how something could be done better, just don't preface your comment with, "Well, back in (blank)..." and try not to do it too terribly often, because it will still carry the same effect. Remember, you are not out there to change the world! Just enjoy that you get to be so lucky to see how things are done differently everywhere and relish the fact that you get paid a good sum of money to travel around and experience the differences in American (and sometimes foreign) culture(s).

Dorothy from Kentucky

Dorothy is an emergency and critical care nurse who places her priorities on benefits and location. She has been traveling for over two years and takes the housing stipend and her RV with her on assignments. She was previously with American Mobile and now travels with Trustaf. Her favorite city has been Lexington, KY.

She had been a nurse for 12 years at the time of her first assignment, so she was fairly comfortable with it. She has enjoyed the nursing staffs everywhere that she had been, and she has made friends that she continues to keep in contact with from every assignment.

She would like to remind a first time traveler to be careful! Your assignment is only as good as your recruiter. Get it in writing and stick to your guns. Adapt to your surroundings, work hard, be a team player, and you will fit in anywhere you go.

Kristi from Texas

Kristi is a surgical nurse who travels for the great salary, benefits and location. She takes the housing stipend and finds her own housing. She has been traveling for over a year and is currently with Talemed. Her favorite city has been Reno, NV.

Her first experience was very nice; however, in the middle of her extended contract her original company merged with National Healthcare and everything went to pot. She got ahold of a horrible recruiter. She had had an excellent recruiter with TVL. Needless to say, the next assignment she switched companies.

She would like to remind newbies to *always get everything in writing*. Companies will promise you the moon to get you to sign with them. Ask the company you are going to work for to have a nurse who already works for them contact you. This way you can ask them personally about their experience. Have a list of questions written down before you start contacting companies. She says, "I have been an OR nurse for 15 yrs. and have had good experiences everywhere I have been. I plan to continue traveling. It is a wonderful way to see the country. I have made so many new friends."

Kristin from Lousiana

Kristin is a critical care nurse who places location and a great recruiter her top priorities. She takes the stipend and spends it on an RV space. In her almost five years of traveling, her favorite city has been Oklahoma City, with Naples, FL and Los Angeles, CA being her least favorites.

She and her husband are both RNs and travel together. Their first assignment was at Emory in Atlanta, GA. It was OK. There was a little reverse racism going on there, but they just minded their own business.

She would like to remind first timers to be very wary of any promises made over the phone. "My recruiter is great and does an excellent job of keeping us out of not traveler friendly areas. The nurse manager of the ICUs at Naples Community completely lied about floating (how often and where). I extended only because I drove all the way from LA and had spent all my savings for the trip so I was stuck. I was floated MANY times to med/surg floors which is very difficult for an ICU RN...read TOO many pts. When you where floated out you received no help, always took the crazy pts, admits etc. Bottom line...talk to other travelers to get the down low."

Rhonda from Florida

Rhonda is a telemetry and step-down nurse who travels for the great salary and different locations. She takes the housing stipend and finds her own housing. She has been traveling for over two years with Fastaff. Her favorite city has been Reno, NV, with Bakersfield, CA being her least favorite.

Her first assignment was a three-week strike and she absolutely loved it. She did a four-week travel assignment next and was hooked. She loves her job as a nurse!

She would like to remind the first timer to ask a lot of questions and get everything in writing. Travel with a buddy the first time. Be flexible at the hospital, smile and work hard. It always pays off! Enjoy yourself; you will meet so many new friends.

Tina from Illinois

Tina is an intensive care and emergency room nurse who places her priorities on a great recruiter and location. She takes the one bedroom housing supplied by Travel Nurse Solutions. In her almost five years of traveling, her worst experience was with On Assignment. Her favorite hospital was in Seattle, WA, with her least favorite being in Providence, RI.

Her first assignment was a disaster; the countryside was great, but the nurses were standoffish, stuck up, snooty, management was disorganized, she didn't get paid for three weeks, if they made a mistake on your check they pulled the entire deposit out of your bank, didn't pay any bounced check fees and left you on your own.

She would like to remind first timers to stay out of the politics. Most of us travel because we don't like the games, so remember that. Keep quiet for a few weeks, watch things, listen and learn who to go to for protocols etc. Not everyone likes travelers.

Bobbye from Mississippi

Bobbye is a telemetry nurse who places her priorities on salary and location. She takes the one bedroom housing paid for by Trinity Healthcare. Her favorite city has been Mesa, AZ.

Her first traveling experience was at Banner Baywood hospital in Mesa, Az. The first thirteen weeks was like a honeymoon. She asked for single housing for her and her husband and they put her up in a three bedroom townhome on a beautiful golf course! The townhome was gorgeous and fully equipped. As far as the hospital goes, they had a nurse patient ratio of 1:5 max and they stuck to it. They had experienced charge nurses that were really helpful. They even had a monitor tech, which I find now not all hospitals have in telemetry. She made a lot of friends there, and she feels it is an excellent hospital.

Her tips for a first timer includes finding another nurse that works for the company you are thinking of working for and grill him/her on the how the company really works!

Juanna from Michigan

Juanna is an intensive care nurse who places travels for the great location as her priority. She has been traveling for under a year with bridge staffing. Her overall experiences haven't been so good with her disaster hospital listed as UCSF in San Francisco, CA.

During her phone interview with the UCSF ICU Nurse Manager she stressed the fact that it was her first travel assignment as well as her first time working in the USA; therefore, she did not want an assignment where floating was involved. The nurse manager confirmed both on the phone and in person that she wouldn't float out of the unit, then she was floated 50% of the time! .

She felt that her license and the patients she cared for were jeopardized on a regular basis. She addressed the issue with the nurse manager who "blackmailed" her into keeping her mouth shut or she would discontinue the contract (with all the financial penalties of housing for thirteen weeks in San Francisco for her to pay for. She would have basically ended up paying to work!) She kept a low profile, fearing what was awaiting her every time she came in to work. She decided to look at it as a challenge. She worked hard and harder and had a lot of positive feedback from her colleagues. The nurse manager of her "home unit" interacted with her a total of five minutes over thirteen weeks. She remained extremely polite and respectful, even though she came all the way from Canada to California based on the nurse manager's lies. Nonetheless, she was "thanked" by this same nurse manager giving a bad reference to her future prospective employers. It was overall a good experience work wise. It pushed her to her limits and she did learn a lot. Her agency gave her the assurance they were backing her up, but they actually didn't take any actions to correct the situation. As many others wrote, everything that is said should be written in the contract. Do not make the same mistake she made by trusting your recruiter/the hospital when they tell you that the contracts are standard and "such thing" (whatever concerns you) will/will not happen. She has heard one too many times the "trust me" sentence, and she was wrong to actually trust them when she knew that she wasn't satisfied with what was (or wasn't) written in the contract. Make sure you can get out of the contract without any financial penalty for you if the experience turns out to be less than satisfactory, and especially if it is disastrous or worse yet, dangerous. It looks like the agency you choose matters less than the recruiter you choose. Make him/her spell out every detail and have it written down in your contract. Many things that were told to her orally by her recruiter did not happen and he later on denied saying it. It could be highly frustrating, and in her case, costly! It might only be thirteen weeks, but it could have major repercussions in your future too, so be extra careful. Protecting your practice and license isn't that easy when you are between the rock and the hard place; you either do your best with what you have (most of the time, without what you actually need) or you just plain refuse the assignment and then you could be accused of endangering your patients by leaving them without a nurse. Both ways, you are stuck. So her best advice is this: avoid any place that could potentially treat you this way, and if it still happens, make sure your contract allows you a way out.

Linda from Tennessee

Linda is a cardiac nurse who places her priorities on a great salary and benefits. She takes the one bedroom paid for by National Healthcare. In her almost five years of traveling, she includes Medstaff Inc. a disaster company, along with Baptist East in Memphis, TN as being her disaster hospital with her least favorite city being Kingsport, TN. Her favorite assignment was in Lebanon, NH.

On her first assignment she had an average of fifteen patients per night in Memphis. It was just awful and she felt like she was stuck in the assignment. She would like to remind a first timer not to compare one place to another. You must be adaptable and let things just roll off your back. Remember, it is only thirteen weeks!

Elizabeth from Michigan

Elizabeth is a home health nurse who places her priorities on salary and benefits. She has been traveling for over six years and is currently with Fastaff.

Her first experience was great. That was what made her decide to keep traveling. The hospital was friendly, along with the staff. She learned lots about travel from listening to other travelers.

She would like to remind travelers to check out the companies before traveling. She got hooked up with Access Nurses. What a disaster! They were to pay for housing, utilities, etc. The hospital cancelled her contract, along with five other travelers for "money" reasons. The hospital then told Access Nurses a different story. The Agency believed the hospital. They left her stranded in California and were not going to give her a paycheck because she did not complete the contract. She had to *beg* to get enough money to fly back to Michigan. Then they sent her a bill for everything they had paid for—housing, housing deposit, utilities, drug screen, etc. The bill was almost $3000.00 and they immediately turned the bill over to a collection agency. They violated the contract by trying to charge her. No one at the agency would take her phone calls, so she had to get an attorney. Lesson learned: *never* work for a company that is going to charge you a fee if your contract is cancelled!

Lena from Florida

Lena is a labor and delivery nurse who places importance on a great recruiter and location. She has been traveling for under a year and takes the one bedroom that is paid for. So far her favorite hospital has been Modesto, CA.

Her first assignment was great. She decided to make a total change and travel across the county. From day one she met fellow travelers and enjoyed doing activities with them. The hospital was great, a very smooth sailing ship. She absolutely loved the hospital!

She would like to remind first timers to get everything in writing, even if they told you one thing on the phone. If it's not in your contract the recruiter will act like it was never said. Research your companies and locations ahead of time and never go with a company if you don't like the recruiter.

Teresa from California

Teresa is also a labor and delivery nurse who travels for the salary and recruiter as her priorities. She takes her RV on assignments with Cross Country TravelCorps. Her favorite hospitals have been Memorial in Modesto, CA and Mt. Sinai in Miami, FL. Her least favorite hospital was Community Hospital of New Port Richey, RI.

Her first experience was in Rugby, ND. She stayed for a year then went back home to finish her BSN. Rugby was a terrific town with friendly people and a great staff. Her hints to first timers include: Research, research, research. Keep your mouth shut for the first few weeks and work your butt off, then you can relax a little. Even though most places are friendly toward travelers, you are still not a staff person, so be very careful about what you say and do.

Brenda from Alabama

Brenda is a long term care nurse who travels for the great salary and even takes the housing stipend. She has been traveling with Nursefinders for a year.

About her first assignment she writes, "I came to Rhode Island as a First Travel Assignment. I worked at the Grand Islander in Middletown. I was accustomed to friendly doctors and nurses. Some of these doctors are rude and never call you back. Most of the staff was great, but a few of the staff were horrible! They bitched and whined about things that I thought were plain trifling! There was one incidence that I got blamed for something and there were several of their staff there that nothing was said to them. My recruiter—I cannot say enough about Jackie! She went above and beyond for me and would go to bat for me in a heartbeat! I shall miss her when my 13 weeks is up! I extended for 1 week and that is it! I will be glad to be home for a few weeks before I hit the road again. All in all, it has been a great learning experience!! I did get a 2 weeks orientation and I *was very* grateful for that."

Her hints to a first timer include reading your contract and when the company that you are being interviewed for interviews you—interview them as well! Keep your eyes and ears open and remember, you are the guest and the home team has the advantage.

Joanne from North Carolina

Joanne is an emergency room nurse who classifies benefits and a great recruiter as her top priorities. She prefers two bedroom housing and doesn't mind paying some for that! She has been traveling for almost five years with Cross Country TravCorps. Her favorite city has been Chapel Hill, NC.

She feels that she has been very blessed in that her first experience was a plus, providing new found friends and a great place to live in Chapel Hill, NC. She would definitely recommend travel nursing!

Joanne would like to tell first timers, "Life can be a great experience if you let it. I'm now in Rocky Mount, NC. This is my second assignment and this is in the area I most love. It's not been easy as I've been here 1.5yrs now. In that I mean the ER here is extremely busy. I've been here long enough to get my nose in the politics of the place (not always the wisest thing to do) and now I'm struggling with moving on. *Oh, boy!*"

Katrina from West Virginia

Katrina is a tele/med/surg nurse who places salary and location number ones on her list. She takes the one bedroom housing from Nurse Choice. She has traveled with Supplemental, but was not happy with them. Her favorite assignments have been in New Orleans, LA, and Prescott Valley, AZ, with her least favorite being in Columbia, SC.

After a ten year layoff she finally got back on the horse in January and had the best first experience in New Orleans. The hospital was very appreciative of the travelers coming to relieve stressed out staff post-Katrina. The housing left something to be desired, but the wonderful people made up for the lack of luxury housing. She liked it so much that she stretched out a four week assignment into five months, and she would like to go back again someday. She will always be grateful to Ochsner Medical Center for making her first experience at traveling a lifetime career memory. She loves NOLA!

Her hints to a first timer include 1) Going the first time with a company that someone you know has recommended to you. 2) You need to read between the lines during the interview; for instance, if they use the word "challenge" this may be a buzzword for something else such as more critical patients than you're used to or high nurse/pt ratio etc. 3) The interview is also your chance to find out about them, so don't forget to ask lots of questions. 4) Read your contract before you sign it. You don't want to get miles away from home and realize something isn't in writing that they promised on the phone.

Angela from South Carolina

Angela is an operating room nurse who has been traveling for almost five years. She places importance on a great salary and benefits. She is currently traveling with Cirrus Medical Staffing after a disaster with First Assist. Her favorite city has been Washington, DC, with Turlock, CA, being her least favorite.

Her first travel experience was at Duke University in Durham, NC. She was close to family for her first assignment, which was very nice. She was going through a painful divorce at the time, and travel nursing gave her the perfect excuse to run away from home. She did not bring my emotional breakdowns to work, although she did come to trust a couple of co-workers enough to tell her sad story. She worked with Vascular/Transplant/General/Oncology surgeons and the Transplant docs were great! The rest were typical arrogant jerks. She wrote her very first complaint about a surgeon, and it turns out that he was the head of the Plastics Dept. Nursing management was incredibly supportive at the time. Overall, the assignment was a great learning experience that was unfortunately overshadowed by her own personal emotional tragedy. It hasn't stopped her though! She still gets goosebumps thinking of all the choices she has for the location of her next assignment! She would like to remind newbies to never lose confident in themselves.

Marilyn from South Carolina

Marilyn is an emergency room nurse who places her priority on a great location. She has been traveling for under a year with Travel Nurse Solutions. The people at Havasu Regional were very friendly, but staffing was a nightmare.

Havasu was her first position and she did renew it. The people, in general, were very friendly and receptive. Almost all staffers were travelers. She loved the area. It is a little tourist town so the hospital gets the regular party goers and lake accidents. All in all, it was a good experience. The staffing could have been much better, but the manager was very amenable.

What would she like to tell first time travelers? "Go for it. I was leery at first, but it has been a great experience. I got to met new people and see new places, although you can't be afraid to do things on your own.

Betty from Arkansas

Betty is a med/surg nurse who travels for the excellent pay rate. She has been traveling for over six years and currently travels with Nationwide Nurse Travel Professionals. Her favorite place was Lake Havasu City, AZ, with her least favorite city being New Jersey.

Her first experience was not bad, just not what she expected. She was new at it and sort of unsure of how it would be as a traveler, but she did ot and she has been traveling ever since.

She would like to remind travelers that it does get easier. She has traveled with a lot of agencies in her six plus years of traveling, but the agency the she is with now is the best so far. They have been able to keep her working and pretty much find a position in the area she wants to be in, or close to it. Betty knows that anytime she has a problem all she has to do is call her recruiter and she will be there to talk and listen or assist her with her problem. They sent her information on the area and maps she was traveling to. She has found them to be honest and upfront about everything and so far she has had no surprises. She feels like she has found her travel nursing home and now she can travel with ease and no worries. Her advice to any new traveler is to be patient and research the area you want to travel to, and even the facility. Talk to your recruiter and ask for information on the area.

Teresa from Illinois

Teresa is a med/surg nurse who is now traveling with Aureus Medical after she was left to find her own housing with Supplemental Healthcare. She places importance on an honest recruiter and a great salary. Her favorite assignment was in St. Petersburg, FL.

Her first assignment was a good experience. She was fortunate to go to a hospital where a friend had just completed an assignment. The friend even met her back at the assignment location and introduced her to some friends from the floor and helped her find her way around some before she went back home. The staff was very friendly and helpful.

She would like to remind travelers to get everything in writing and save all emails. You never know when you will need the information. She found that one out first hand. Don't back down, and be strong. It is a good experience and can teach you not only about nursing but about yourself too.

Krista from Kansas

Krista is an operating nurse who travels for the great benefits and locations. She has been traveling with American Mobile for almost two years, and takes the two bedroom paid for housing. Her favorite city was San Diego, CA.

She traveled a couple of years ago and loved it. She only did it for 6 months. Now her kids are out of high school and, being divorced now, she is free to travel. She is now on her first assignment this time around. She was welcomed by the staff/ mgmt/housekeeping/biomed... "Everyone here has been so nice!" she says. The case load is manageable too. The other travelers here have taught her loads and she hopes to pass on that knowledge when she can.

She would like to remind other travelers to always, always get everything in writing. More important than the company you work for is the recruiter that works for you! A good recruiter makes or breaks the deal. She loves her recruiter now.

Winnie from South Carolina

Winnie is a telemetry nurse who places the most importance on a great recruiter and excellent salary. She is currently with MedFirst Staffing, but she is looking for something better. After almost five years of traveling, her favorite assignment has been in Anderson, SC, with her least favorite in Chapel Hill, SC.

Her first travel experience was a phychiatric job at the state hospital. She was treated like family, like part of the team. There was little difference between contract and "full timers." They were great people, and backed you up when things could/and would get hairy.

She would tell first timers, "If you don't have it in your contract, you won't have it. Think things through, get it in writing, and *make sure* you have an out. Some agencies will stick you will everything, and it *may not* be your fault.

Tina from Maine

Tina is a telemetry and PACU nurse who travels for the great salary and location, along with a wonderful recruiter. She has been traveling for over ten years and is currently with Professional Respiratory Care Services after a terrible experience with Cross Country TravCorp. Her favorite hospital was in Phoenix, AZ, with her least favorite being Los Angeles, CA and Brockton Hospital in Brockton, MA.

Her first travel assignment with Cross Country was a total nightmare. The job was less than great, but the company was the worst. It took more than three weeks to get her pathetic paycheck of less than $350 a week. Daily attempts to reach a recruiter were answered about every sixth call. Also, being new, they really knew how to intimidate her into feeling that she had no other options. Thank God she spoke with Andy from PPR, who made her realize not all companies are heartless. All subsequent companies have been reasonable and workable.

She would like to tell the newbies that no matter where you are, you can learn. It is OK to bring new ideas, but don't complain about how everything is done. Different is good, that is why you travel. Also, don't get sucked in to any of the gossip. Work hard first, feel out the staff and situation, and then you can relax a little. As for your company, your nursing recruiter can't fix your daily assignment so don't call every day to complain. Cry wolf and the important issues won't be taken seriously. Most importantly, your license is your career, so if it is truly unsafe *you can* get out. Don't be threatened or bullied. Remember, it's supposed to be fun.

Christine from Nebraska

Christine is an emergency and intensive care nurse who also has experience as a house supervisor. She travels for the location and salary with Aureus Medical. She has been traveling for almost two years, with her favorite hospital being Grand Island, Nebraska.

She did a total of three contracts in Sidney, Nebraska at a small Critical Access Hospital. She was able to do everything: ER, CICU, Med/Surg, Outpatients, and Swing Bed. It was a great experience and the staff, for the most part, was awesome. It was harder to leave there than it was to leave the hospital she left to travel where she had worked for twenty-four years.

Her suggestions to newbies include: 1) Research companies. 2) Ask more questions and 3) Talk to other Travelers.

Tarrah from California

Tarrah is a Med/Surg and Oncology nurse who places her important factors as salary and location. She takes the standard one bedroom housing paid for by Nurses in Partnership. Her favorite city has been Los Angeles, CA, with her least favorite assignment at Century City Doctor's Hospital.

She is still in it and while she loves Los Angeles and loves living in Beverly Hills, her company, Nurses in Partnership, and the hospital were not honest while recruiting her. All the nurses there are travelers and hate it, counting down the days to leave. There *is no* director of nursing or protocols to follow. To make things worse, she feels like her company hasn't been paying accurately and can't account for money that is owed to her.

She would like to remind beginning traveling nurses to do a lot of research. Please talk to other travelers about do's and don'ts, and get everything in writing in your contract. Be specific about it. Have a good recruiter; if you aren't comfortable during the recruiting process, look elsewhere.

Lacy from Mississippi

Lacy is an ER nurse who places her priorities on a great location with a wonderful recruiter. She takes the standard one bedroom housing and travels now with Travel Nurse Solutions. Her favorite assignment was her first assignment in Memphis, TN.

She is currently working at Methodist Hospital in Memphis, TN, and she says "It's awesome. The computerized charting in the emergency department is something that has taken some getting used to, but everyone is super nice." She would recommend this facility to anyone. They care about their travelers and are always asking her if she's being treated ok. She loves her company, TNS. Her recruiter, Chris Woodham, is *awesome*.

She would like to remind all newbies to make sure to do their homework about a facility and town. Make sure to look up information about each hospital that they are told about by her recruiter. And mapquest is a lifesaver.

Bonita from Virginia

Bonita is a telemetry nurse who travels for the great benefits and locations. She has been traveling for over two years and takes the standard one bedroom housing. She travels now with Clinical One after a problem with Medstaff. Her favorite assignment was in Las Vegas, NV, with her least favorite being in New Orleans, LA.

Her first travel assignment was with a great little hospital in Inverness, Fla. The staff was a very traveler- friendly staff. She floated in turn and went all over the hospital. It was a 165 bed hospital, run by the community drs., so the bottom line was what was good for the patients.

Her advice to a first timer would be to be flexible and remember even the worst assignment is only for thirteen weeks, and the best assignments can last as long as you want (usually).

Charlotte from Mississippi

Charlotte is a perioperative and critical care nurse who places importance on a great salary and benefits. She takes the housing stipend and travels in an RV. She has been traveling for under a year with Travel Nurse Across America. Her favorite assignment was in Hanford, CA, with her least favorite being Deming, NM.

Her first assignment was wonderful—very traveler friendly and well organized All personnel that she worked with went out of their way to make her feel welcomed and at home. It was hard to leave after the six month mark.

She would like to remind traveling nurses to be cautious, professional, and take care with your duties. Remember to nurse as any prudent nurse would and give your patients the care that you would desire for yourself and your family members.

Abbie from Pennsylvania

Abbie is a med/surg/tele nurse who places her priorities on a great salary and benefits. She has been traveling for under a year with Nightingale and is happy with them. She doesn't have a favorite or disaster city—yet.

Her first assignment consisted of no rental car reimbursement; the recruiter thought she would take the bus, which would mean walking one mile and one and a half hours to catch the bus. She rented a car, at her expense, for $600 a month. She lived in an apartment complex that wasn't safe and went to a hospital in unsafe area. It was a very scary time for her in Phoenix. On top of that, the company only paid up to $100 for utilities and the electric alone was $180 a month. She lost quite a bit of money on that assignment.

She would like to remind traveling nurses not to sign anything until you have everything covered such items as car rental and utilities.

Jade from Florida

Jade is a med/surg/tele and wound care nurse who places priorities on a company with great salary and benefits with a lot of great locations. She has been traveling with Nightingale, but is ready for a change. Although she has a lot of nice places that she has been to, Glendale, AZ, was not one of them!

On her first assignment the recruiter told her everything that she wanted to hear, but did not carry through with very many of the promises. The recruiter got her 2200 miles away from her home, and forgot about her the minute she got her commission. Jade felt stuck and lonely. She had to fight for every dime they had promised to reimburse her. The recruiter also was very unavailable on the phone. Jade is grateful to have found another traveler in the apartment complex. Even though she felt that her apartment complex and hospital were in an unsafe area, she loved the people she worked with. It was filled with travelers. It was kind of hard, though, as they were all from different nations. The first assignment is the hardest and the one that you learn the most from. When her first paycheck was over $1,000 short, she started to cry.

Her advice to a first time traveler would be to get everything discussed in writing. If you don't, they will tell you, "That's not in your contract," even though you know you talked about it and they promised it to you. Do your homework on the hospital and the area. Bring a laptop, cell phone, at least ten uniform sets, items from home, and things to keep you busy on your off-time. It gets lonely. Read the newspaper and find out from locals what there is to do in the area. Make sure you know whether or not you are to bring items from home for your apt. or if it is fully furnished with kitchen items, etc. It gets expensive to buy these things. Locate the nearest Goodwill if you have to, and make sure that you have at least $1000 for extras to make up for what "errors" there may be or for what you need to buy that you forgot.

Denise from Ohio

Denise works med/surg/tele through Rn Demand, after a disastrous experience from Liquid Agents. Her favorite city has been Laguna Beach, CA, with her least favorite being Hurricane, WV where it was a horrible hospital, but the town wasn't too bad. She has been traveling for almost five years and takes the standard one bedroom housing.

Her first travel experience was all about location, location, location! Roy Lester Schneider Hospital, St Thomas, USVI. She loved the island. She snorkeled every day (except when hurricane Jean hit them), swam, etc. She loved her apartment at Sapphire Village Balcony view—nothing but ocean. All of the travel nurses were nice. Everybody helped each other out. They even bought each other food when their pay didn't clear or they lost a debit card or the hospital didn't get it faxed on time, (You know...*Island* time not US mainland time...and the hospital faxed/verified...we didn't) The hospital was grossly understaffed (1:11 Nurse/Pt ratio *with no* nursing assistant was not uncommon). Supplies? Forget it honey! The only IV pumps were 20+ years old, only used for heparin or other hi risk drips (if you found a pump at all and if you could find tubing for the pumps). She once gave her lunch to a diabetic patient who had no food. But forget the hospital. She felt like the eight weeks of hardship was worth spending time on the Island.

What would she like to tell a first timer? "Before you travel with a company always look them up in the travel nurse online forums (Delphi, highwayhypodermics.com, and ultimatenurse.com, etc) If there are a lot of nurses who report satisfaction with them, leave them on your list. If there are a lot of bad experiences with an agency, drop them like a hot potato! A leopard does not change its spots. And list what's important to you. Her list includes: 1. Housing, private. She doesn't share housing with strangers. Everything paid for, *all* utilities (including local phone and basic cable). Housing should be completely furnished, right on down to pots/pans. She refused to go schlepping her household goods all over the country. 2. Day one benefits with dependant coverage available at a reasonable price. 3. Weekly pay, direct deposit, etc. (Make up your own list.) Stick to your list; she always get everything she asked for. Well, she hopes that helps. Buena Suerta!

Kathryn from Wisconsin

Kathryn is a rehab and medical nurse who prefers to have a great recruiter and salary over benefits and location. She currently travels with Emerald Healthcare, after a horrible experience from RTG Medical. Her favorite city has been San Rafael, CA, with her least favorite being Chico, CA, and Enloe Medical Center.

Her first travel assignment was horrible. Her company gave her the wrong directions. The staff treated her worse than dirt. Her company wouldn't stand behind her when the hospital tried to discriminate and harass her. Her company stranded her three hours from home when she wouldn't renew with them. They placed her in an apartment that needed constant maintenance in that the toilet and tub kept backing up. They charged her for items that they were supposed to pay for, even though it was agreed upon in the written contract that they would pay for these items. They placed her into a contract with another hospital without my authorization and then blamed her when it had to be cancelled because she did not renew with them. She really felt that RTG was only out to make a buck and did not care about its travelers.

She would like to remind first timers to ask around for references. Ask if there are other travelers that can give a reference for the company. Visit several travel nursing forums and other traveling nursing websites to see what you need to include in the contract and if the hospital has been listed as being a horrible hospital, etc.

Jill from Florida

Jill is an ER nurse who places salary and benefits as her top priorities. She has been traveling under a year with PPR Travel.

Her first travel job was at Northside Hospital in St. Petersburg, Florida. It was a seventeen bed emergency room in which the staff was very friendly. Nurse/patient ratio was hard at times, being six to one, but when you went to the charge nurse and told them you would take no more, they would listen. All in all it was tolerable for thirteen weeks.

She would like to remind first timers to be very flexible. Get some experience before you start. They expect travelers to come in and need very little instruction. Always keep a sense of humor. Also smile a lot. You only have to put up with where you are for thirteen weeks, unlike the full time staff that are there year after year.

Joan from North Carolina

Joan is a labor and delivery nurse who places location and benefits as her reasons for traveling. She has been traveling for under a year with Bridgestaffing. Her favorite city has been Richmond, VA.

This was her first travel assignment experience, and she felt like she made the right decision to quit her job of 16 years and start traveling. Chippenham Johnston Willis Hospital L&D department in Richmond, VA made her first assignment a very positive experience. They asked her to take another assignment and she resigned another eight-week contract because of the staff and doctors that she worked with. She felt like she had made lasting friendships and she was sad to leave Richmond, VA, but she looked forward to expanding her travel career that she had started.

She would like to remind first timers to do their homework and decide what is most important to them as salary, benefits, etc. before signing a contract.

Eileen from Washington

Eileen is an OB nurse who places salary and a great recruiter as her top priorities. She takes the two bedroom housing provided by the Quest Group and has been traveling for almost five years. Her favorite assignment was in Oak Harbor, WA at the Naval Hospital, with her least favorite being Centralia, WA.

Her first traveling experience was awful! There were nurses who were rude and basically mean to her. The charge nurses dumped their patients on her and she went back and the charge nurse slept until six in the morning then blamed her for not charting on her patients! She told her she'd already assessed and charted on them. The nurse manager was very rude. She even had two of the worst deliveries of her career at the hospital—both on the same night!

She would like to remind first timers to remember that they are a guest at the hospital where they are assigned. Act in a professional, polite manner. Know your skill level and limitations and be honest and up front about it. Know that you will learn something new from every hospital you work at. Look at each new assignment in that light, and don't try to go in and tell the place how it should be run or find fault continuously. That is one huge mistake she finds travelers do too frequently. It makes the staff dislike you. Look to learn from them, but know what the standards of care are and follow them. Also, realize that you will be watched closely at first in most places until the staff is sure of you and your skills. Stand up for your patients—and yourself. Don't let them dump on you, but don't sit on your butt and read a magazine when the rest of the staff is running either. Watch the other staff and see what they do that maybe they haven't told you about. Buy a clear plastic badge holder to wear with your name badge and place a card in it that contains all the most frequently needed phone numbers you will likely need on the spur of the moment. For example, she works L&D so she put the docs contact numbers on my badge, the supervisor's number, the other areas of the unit's phone numbers. This allows her to know exactly where the number is when she needs it. It saves time when in a hurry. If you don't have a recruiter who works for you to iron out the problems that are sure to arise during a contract, then find one who will. That doesn't mean you have to leave the company, but you might have to ask for a new recruiter. Get a good tax advisor. Track all your mileage, keep good records. Pack light. Most of all, *have fun!*

Kay from Missouri

Kay is an emergency room nurse who travels for the great salary and benefits. She has been traveling for over a year now, with her favorite city being Tucson, AZ.

At her first assignment the hospital staff was mostly nice, except for one vicious physician and tech. The patients and staff were primarily Spanish-speaking. She was in a dangerous area of town, dangerous staff/patient ratios, and an insecure working environment. Luckily, she had a good company, a good recruiter, a nice apartment and her husband to keep her sane. Even with the nice staff she would not return to this facility unless the safety issue was addressed first.

She would like to remind first timers not to go until you are competent in the area you are presenting yourself for and to have a backup plan if the contract or company falls through, and have some backup cash. Don't take anything personal and expect bumps in the plan with pay/housing/hospital etc. Do not expect orientation; they expect you to work without it.

Steve from Ohio

Steve is an intensive care nurse who places salary and location as his top priorities. He takes the one bedroom option, paid for from Professional Respiratory Care Services. He once traveled with World Health, but never again. His favorite place was San Francisco, with his least favorite assignment being Summerlin Medical and Las Vegas, NV.

He had a great first time experience in Arizona in an MICU. The staff was incredibly friendly and management treated travelers like staff. It gave him a great taste about traveling.

His hints for a first time traveler? "Before you take your 1st assignment you must evaluate what is important to you, i.e. money, location, housing, benefits and don't sacrifice the important ones. There are many companies out there. Be sure to interview the hospital management before excepting to get an idea of the unit/hospital and expectations..."

W.C. from Ohio

W.C. is a critical care nurse who travels for the great benefits, salary and location. He has been traveling for almost two years now and finds his own housing. This traveler is currently with On Assignment, but would change companies if something better came along. Their favorite city has been Richmond, VA, with Providence, RI being their least favorite.

Their first time experience was great! It was a small hospital in Weirton, WV. They had excellent staffing, and WC worked both telemetry and the cardiac care unit for six months. It was very traveler-friendly, and really set her views on traveling as something she will do for a long time!

Her pointers for first timers include: Not getting involved with all the hospital politics, keep smiling, help the other staff but remember who helps you also! Never compromise your nursing values, no matter what. Stand your ground and fight for what you believe in. Always research the company you are considering working for, as well as the hospital you are considering traveling to and above all, *always always* get everything in writing, no matter how nice the recruiter or company sounds. In closing, just remember the golden rule: Do unto others as you would have them do unto you!! Good luck, and have fun!

Chris from New York

Chris is a surgical technologist who travels for the love of money, benefits, location, and recruiter. He takes the two bedroom housing from Preferred Healthcare. He has been traveling for almost two years. His favorite assignments have been San Jose, San Francisco, and Palto Alto because of the beautiful weather. Most of the assignments have been good, with the worst being UCSF-San Francisco.

He was scared and paranoid all the time, knowing that he didn't know anyone in California. He felt home sick for several days; however, it was kind of cool because he learned to be independent and know himself better. Also, traveling is the wisest decision he has ever made.

What would he like to tell first time travelers? "You'll meet very cool travelers and you will always look out for each other. Referring only to travelers! You will be able to discover certain cities that you have never been to. It is pretty exciting! Although, for first time travelers, please do not let any recruiter fool you. Please do a lot of research with any travel nursing company. Hmm, also kind of make your own list of all the things that you want within your company before signing any contracts. Ask as many questions as you want and if you feel can't get any answer to your question, then drop that company ASAP!"

Gloria from Florida

Gloria works in the emergency room and has been traveling for over six years. She places her priorities on a great recruiter and salary. She takes the one bedroom paid for by Nationwide Nurses. She loved the Southwest and Arizona, but hated Nebraska.

She had her first travel experience with Nationwide Nurses and they will have her last until she retires. She did try two other travel companies in between assignments, not because she was not happy with Nationwide but because she really wanted a state they did not have much in, and oh man, what a mistake! She won't name any names, but the travel experience was horrible—with both other companies, actually! She went back to Nationwide Nurses and it has been smooth sailing. Her recruiter is Aawesome! She calls her back if she ever needs her and most of the time can get right through to her. The housing is the best and she even takes her dogs!

She would like to remind first timers to be honest and open with what you want, ask questions, and be sure to tell your agency any worries or concerns you have.

Michele from Oklahoma

Michele is an intensive care nurse who places salary and benefits as her top priorities, with a great recruiter and excellent location next. She takes the two bedrooms paid for and has been traveling for almost five years. She is currently with Medical Express, after a disastrous experience with Premier Healthcare. Her least favorite assignments were in Oakland, CA and Hopewell, VA, with Tucson, AZ her favorite.

With her first assignment, her recruiter was wonderful! It was a challenge for her to leave her home and live on the road. If asked to do it again, she would in a heartbeat!

She would like to remind first timers to listen to seasoned travelers...they have the experience on how to deal with companies, situations, and a lousy travel job. If you are not flexible and are not able to pick up new things quickly, it's not time yet for you. Always hook up with other travelers to hang out with when you're in a new city/town.

Gay from Louisiana

Gay is a PACU nurse who has been traveling for almost five years. She is currently traveling with Cross Country TravCorp, but would consider another company. Her favorite city has been Albuquerque, NM.

Her first assignment was at Memorial in Modesto, CA. Everyone was very friendly. They were especially sweet since she had just been through Katrina. The job was easy, compared to the work of her pre travel job.

She would like to remind the newbies to go in with a good attitude. Be happy. It makes the staff feel good and they respond in a friendly manner. You also get good evaluations when they like you. Just don't sweat the small stuff, although she thinks that this is easier said because she works PACU. You would never have more than two pts at a time in any reputable hospital. She thinks that other units could be much more difficult to travel to.

Emily from Michigan

Emily is a labor and delivery nurse who travels for the great salary, but always wants a great recruiter. She has been traveling for almost two years with Nova Pro. Her favorite city has been Denver, CO, with Reno, NV, being her least favorite.

Her first travel experience was in Denver at Exempla Lutheran. This was a great hospital and very friendly to travelers. My experience in Reno Nevada...well, lets just say she probably would not have chosen this hospital had she interviewed with the actual unit instead of her company and if she had been given the correct information.

She would like to remind new travelers that if you have found a good travel company and have started the interviewing process, please try to interview with the unit itself. She has found that if the travel company interviews you they may have information about the unit that is either old, wrong, or hasn't been updated.

Sometimes this information can determine whether or not you choose the hospital.

Jasmin from Florida

Jasmin is a critical/intensive care and PACU nurse who places money and location as very important to her, with benefits and a great recruiter ranking next. She takes the housing stipend as she travels with HRN Services. Her favorite city has been San Francisco.

She enjoyed her first travel assignment. She says, "If you're flexible, if you're outgoing, and you value teamwork, you're not going to be upset with travelers always floating, having the worst patients, etc. She had a great agency and great recruiter.

Her advice to first timers would include: Don't always go with the bigger companies, such as American Mobile, Cross Country, etc. There are some great mid-size to smaller companies. As a first time traveler, traveling to San Fran by herself, HRN provided her a great package. If she did ever get bored, she would always be able to pick up an extra shift at the hospital she was assigned to or they would provide other per diem at a same day surgery, school of dentistry, etc. Higher hourly wages does not always mean you're going to get the most out of your pay stub. Look at the whole package.

Mary from Arizona

Mary is a PICU nurse who travels mainly for a great location and top salary, followed by benefits and a great recruiter. She takes the one bedroom that is paid for by RN Network. She had a horrible experience with AMN Healthcare. Her favorite assignment was in Salt Lake City, with Indianapolis being her least favorite. Her assignment at the University of Virginia, Charlottesville, was a disaster.

Her first assignment was in San Diego, CA in 1989. She had a great experience, both at work and off work. She stayed 6 months and only experienced one earthquake!

She would like to remind first timers to take one third of what you think you will need. Do remember to take a few things that will help with homesickness... "I don't care how old you are, a little something familiar is comforting on those odd blue' days. Also, before you go, practice eating at restaurants and going to movies alone," she suggests.

Margaret from California

Margaret is an NICU nurse who places her priorities on a great salary and terrific recruiter. She takes the stipend and finds her own housing. She has been traveling for under a year. She was with Preferred Healthcare, but having a rough time, she switched to Procel. Her favorite assignment was in Irvine, CA, with her least favorite being in Long Beach, CA.

She says that it was wonderful! I started at Irvine Regional Hospital—a small, close-knit facility. She was welcomed by management and staff nurses alike. They patiently answered all of her questions and there was always someone around to help if needed. The equipment may not be the most up-to-date, but it was well-maintained and suits the purpose. Ancillary staff and volunteers were very nice and helpful. There didn't seem to be an overwhelming amount of policies and procedures to worry about, but she didn't feel as though someone was waiting just around the corner to write her up.

She would like to remind first timers, "Get everything in writing! Just as the saying 'If it isn't charted then it wasn't done' applies to a legal case, 'If it isn't in the contract then it isn't guaranteed' applies to the assignment. Enjoy your assignment! Have fun in whatever city you're assigned to. You're only there for up to 13 weeks; go with the flow, don't try to change anything, and for goodness sake, stay out of the politics! Don't worry if others don't like you or resent the fact that you make more money. If they want to make the same general wages, then they can apply to a travel agency just like you did."

Jim from South Carolina

Jim is a med/surg, renal, orthopedics, and oncology nurse who places his priorities on a great recruiter and top salary. He takes the two bedroom that Trinity Healthcare pays for. His favorite city has been Greenville, NC, with Fayetteville, NC being his least favorite.

His first experience at Roper of Charleston, SC was scary. He had to take the PBDS test and was told that if he didn't make it the contract will be canceled. His recruiter was very supportive and had housing ready, even before he took the test. The nurse manager was very hard to deal with, asking him what his dream schedule was and then giving him the exact opposite. He "got" to work every Friday, Saturday, and Sunday for two months. When he talked to the nurse manager, she said, "You are a traveler and very expensive. My core staff is more important, so they get their schedule first." On top of that, she cut his contract early, which was Godsend, and a neurology unit hired him where he had a very nice experience.

His hints to a first timer include: Be flexible. If bad things happen during your thirteen-week contract, suck it in and enjoy going around. Have friends; they make your life less miserable. Research the place and hospital before asking your recruiter to submit you. Also, ask your recruiter if they sent anyone to that place before. Good luck and have fun!

Deb in Indiana

Deb is a critical care nurse who places location as her top priority, followed by salary, benefits, and a great recruiter. She takes the one bedroom paid housing and has been traveling for almost two years. She is currently traveling with AMN Healthcare, after a horrible experience with Cirrus Medical. Her favorite city has been San Diego, with Philadelphia being her least favorite.

She had spoken to many travelers prior to entering traveling. Her first assignment was listed as D/N and she had no idea what that meant and her recruiter brushed over it. Once she arrived at the hospital she was informed that it was rotating shifts. Live and learn! The assignment was fine and she especially enjoyed floating, as the units she floated to were so much nicer than the one to which she was assigned. She renewed three times and hated to leave.

She would like to remind first timers not to over-pack. It took her a few assignments to streamline her packing. She had to throw so much away from her first two assignments that she finally got her act together. She has a flatscreen television, Wii, laptop, two pairs of shoes, uniforms, a small suitcase and file folders with all of her paperwork. If she need things she buys them when she gets there. It is so much easier to buy there than it is to pack it.

Karen from Idaho

Karen is a med/surg/ortho nurse who places benefits and a great recruiter as her top priorities. She takes the one bedroom housing that Travel Nurse Solutions provides. She once traveled with O'Grady Peyton, but never again! Her favorite town has been Columbia, MO, with Phoenix, AZ being her least favorite.

Her first time experience was very nice, at her home state in a small town with great people who were glad to have her there.

Her advice to a first timer would include: If you need good insurance, try to get all the details before you make the decision to go with any particular company. Some have really crappy insurance plans, others have excellent ones.

June from North Carolina

June is a labor and delivery nurse who travels for the salary and great location, followed by benefits and a great recruiter. She has been traveling for under a year and takes the housing stipend. She has been traveling the Premier Healthcare Professional, with her favorite city being Jacksonville, NC.

Her first travel experience was at Onslow Memorial in Jacksonville for five months, and she loved it. The nurses worked well as a team and were friendly to travelers. They treated her like family, which is why she stayed for three contracts. Labor and delivery was busy, but staffing was pretty good for the most part. Some of the doctors were a pain, but that's anywhere you go. Although there were a lot of inductions and epidurals, they had an awesome anesthesia staff. It seemed like they did a lot of C-sections. Although they still had a paper charter, it was a very good place to work.

Her hints to a first timer would include: Stay out of the hospital politics at all costs! She kept on having to learn that one! Maybe extend once, but then move on. She stayed so long that it was hard to say goodbye, and that isn't good when you're a traveler!

Debbie from Virginia

Debbie is a labor and delivery nurse who places her priorities on a great salary and benefits. She travels in her RV with American Mobile. At one time she was with Nova Pro, but never again! Her favorite assignment was in Alexandria, VA, with Sentara Norfolk General Hospital being her worst assignment.

She worked in a fairly new hospital with a new staff, so it was difficult coming in as a traveler and the most experienced nurse most nights she worked; however, the nurses were welcoming and so happy to have her there and worked so well together and with her. The doctors were unhappy and difficult because they were used to working with an inexperienced staff. She enjoyed her time there, but she was happy to leave and move on to a place where she felt she could learn something new and not be the one teaching.

She would like to remind newbies not to get involved in the politics, gossip, etc. Keep your mouth shut and your mind open if you hear staff complaining about the facility or each other. *Smile* constantly. Insist on respect from the doctors, introduce yourself and tell them your credentials and years of experience. Be ready to hit the floor running. Don't complain, but don't let anyone complain about you either! You can be a breath of fresh air for a staff that is overworked and stressed, so have fun and enjoy meeting new people and having new experiences.

Chapter Eighteen

Travel Company Profiles

Top Ten Things to Look For In A Travel Company

There are hundreds of travel companies out there, but the big question becomes "Which is the best one for me?" After reading this article, take the time to make a list of which of these are the top five things you are looking for in a company and let that be your guide down the path to a successful travel company search.

1. Does the company provide adequate health insurance? There are so many types of insurance out there. There are co-payments that range from $10 to $50. Make sure you know exactly what kind of insurance you are getting and that it is worth the money.

2. Does the company provide health insurance within the first 30 days of employment? Some companies still have insurance that begins after 90 days of employment. This saves the company a lot of money because it doesn't become effective until the end of your contract, and if you aren't going to renew your contract or do another contract with that company you will not be covered at all during your assignment.

3. What kind of housing package do they offer? Some companies give you only a one bedroom with electricity while others will help you out with cable, phone, and Internet. Some companies will provide a "soft package" of linens, cookware,

dishes, and other usual living items. Make sure you know exactly what you are getting and exactly what you need.

4. Does the company pay for all pre-employment screening? That should be a given, but you'd be amazed at the ones I find that do not pay for drug screens and physicals. If it's required for you to have such things, the company should pay for it.

5. Does the company provide a 401K with some company match? If the company does not provide 401K with company match you might as well get your own IRA and have full control of your financial future and make your own decisions on what funds you want to invest in. If there is a company match, it is usually worthwhile to make a decision from what the company offers, since they will add in some funds.

6. Does the company offer pay rates over $30? Unless you have a lot of extra perks or you're in the southern resort area, there is no reason why you shouldn't make at least $30 an hour.

7. Does the company offer weekly pay checks that can be directly deposited? I know of a few companies out there that are still sending pay checks by FedEx or courier. Unless you have a nationwide bank, that can be a big pain.

8. Does the company offer the choice to participate in a traveler's advantage program? Although some travelers would rather not take it, it's a great way to put some money into your pocket. Either way, it should be you and your tax advisor's decision as to whether or not to take the tax advantage.

9. Does the company have a plan if there is a missed paycheck? Payroll is human and mistakes are made. The big question is how do they make up for those mistakes? Another nice thing is if they call you if they do not get your time card or if your paycheck is just delayed a week. This is not a have-to for a travel company, but it is the mark of a great company concerned about traveler service.

10. Are missed days either made up or do you have up to three days that are excused. Does the company charge for "assignment expenses" for days missed? With my first company, I missed a day and not only lost a day's wages, but then I was charged by the company for the money that they were out because of the missed

day. It was like missing a day and a half of work. Make sure that you can make up the days before the end of the contract, or that days are excused.

Great companies are not hard to find; you just have to do some shopping around. Below you will find the profiles that were submitted for each company. After reading through these, you can also browse through the Ultimate List of Travel Company Benefits at our updated website: www.highwayhypodermics.com

~*~

8 North Staffing

8 North Staffing has approximately 2000 career opportunities in Alaska, Hawaii, and the Continental U.S. Positions include permanent placements, travel, and per diem assignments, all of which are showcased on their website. After discovering the right assignment, they can have you there in a matter of hours. Rest assured that you 8 North personal assistant will work closely with you every step of the way.

8 North Staffing is a small, but well-connected company. Their personal assistants specialize by geographic regions and are limited to the number of travelers they serve to ensure high levels of personal service. Travelers typically bond with our staff and continue personal relationships even after an assignment is complete.

Their business is based on the principle that "It's all about you." Their *travelers are* their customers and they pride themselves in customizing benefits, housing, travel, etc. to meet individual needs of the traveling nurse. They even provide service to nurses twenty-four hours a day, seven days a week, three hundred and sixty-five days a year. All of their personal assistants provide their cell and home numbers to their travelers and welcome the opportunity to serve.

8 North provides all the benefits that travelers expect...e.g. free professional insurance, free medical insurance, discount health

care, custom tailored housing, transportation reimbursement, referral bonuses, *plus* special benefits like a matching Health Savings Account which can be opened at the *bank you* want. Their professional insurance provides up to $3,000,000 in coverage. Virtually all of their nurses rely solely on their insurance.

Any organization is only as good as its people. The professionals at 8 North share a passion for excellence which translates into a caring environment that puts our travelers first. The ability to match travelers with *the right* position is their "sweet spot." When married with their service ethic, they provide a relationship that is tough to beat. 8 North is also a good corporate citizen, and they offer a unique fund raising opportunity for nursing colleges across the nation. *For every* alumnus that completes a 13-week travel nursing assignment, 8 North will contribute $500 to his or her alma mater for scholarships, capital equipment, etc. The program is clearly a win for all. Alumni are exposed to attractive employment options and the chance to give back to their college, and the nursing school creates a unique, turnkey, fund raising opportunity linked to the professional success of its graduates.

To learn more, please feel free to call them toll free at 1-866-950-5566 or visit them at www.8northstaffing.com. They also can be found at 6090 East Fulton, Ada, MI 49301. Remember, it's all about you!

~*~

Across America Medical Staffing

Across America Med Staffing offers diversity for opportunities travel—short and long term—part time travelers with hours less than 36. This includes perm positions and travel for RNS, ST, CVORT, Cath Lab, Radiology and Allied division professionals. AAMS currently covers 35 states and is growing. They do not make placements out of the United States at the present. Nurses that are ready to go have been placed within the first week they were hired. On an average, from application to job, it takes two weeks or less; for some it's even faster!

Their company is considered small-to-medium, and in AAMS everybody knows your name. You can call your recruiter directly and there are always alternative numbers where someone is available. "I personally have had phone calls at 12-1 a.m. in the morning and have handled the issues. People know they can call," one recruiter says.

AAMS offers one-on-one service with their recruiter. Each recruiter in their company has a direct number that makes it possible for their travelers to speak directly with their people 7 days a week. Even on weekends, they have contact with their personal recruiters. Their housing department manager takes each and every person's need into consideration and offers personalized service. Their administrator is available to answer questions on everything from payroll, 401K to insurance, Monday through Friday. Their clinical support manager is available 7 days a week. They take nursing personally.

AAMS offers Blue Cross/Blue Shield, available within less than 30 days. They cover domestic partners, spouses and children. They offer free health care, as well as 8 different plans to suit the traveler's personal needs. In addition, they have dental, discount vision and life insurance. For those that want additional coverage, they provide AFLAC disability and a 401K, with up to 25% matching available after your first assignment.

What makes them different from many other companies? They listen to what their travelers need. Each person gets personalized service and they will work to develop what they need for themselves and their family. AAMS is about the traveler and their needs; they come first. They pride their nurses in caring about each and every person traveling under their name. AAMS acts as a team, and a team works together to resolve all issues at hand, both the good and the not-so-good.

All of the staff of AAMS combined has over 100 years of experience in the industry. In the last 4 years that they have been in business they have grown as a family and as a company, together with their nurses. Their travelers are the backbone of their company and many have been with them 2-4 years. They are proud of what they have done for their travelers and are highly appreciated. With AAMS their clients are always #1.

Across America Medical Staffing is located at 201 S. Lake Ave., #409, Pasadena, CA 91101. They can be reached by phone at 800-706-6620, and their website can be found at www.acrossamer.com.

~*~

Adex Medical Staffing

Adex Medical Staffing has nationwide travel assignments for specialty RNs, respiratory therapists, and radiology technicians. They have personalized service 24 hours a day, 7 days a week, and they can have you ready to go in one to two weeks. They are a small company that is very personal with their nurses/therapists. The nurses have their recruiter's cell phone number and can call anytime.

Benefits include per diem money, housing, travel expense, medical and dental. They cover the professional liability insurance. The employees are W-2; they do not require additional insurance.

Adex Medical is honest and they follow through with what they tell the nurse they will do. They are always available for the nurses and they pride themselves on building a personal relationship with each one. They know their facilities and try whenever possible to visit them in person.

For more information you can contact them at 1035 Windward Ridge Pkwy, Alpharetta, GA 30005. You can phone them at 866-341-2339. Their website can be found at www.adexmedicalstaffing.com.

~*~

Aedon Staffing

At Aedon, they've developed a comprehensive set of guidelines for evaluating both their company and their applicants so they can refer the right person for the right job at the right time. They also have local staffing, which comprises of highly-skilled dependable staff for short-term needs, such as coverage for sick days, holidays, evenings, weekend shifts, scheduled leaves of absence and peak census times. Their travel staff is professional and flexible to alleviate long-term staffing shortages by committing to work with you for 13 weeks or more at any location. Their temporary to permanent staff program is a risk-free employment method that allows both their company and the employee the opportunity to "test" the job before making a permanent commitment. Their permanent staffing option is a reliable, qualified staff to fill permanent positions within the medical facility. They bring together the premier healthcare providers with first-rate healthcare professionals, including, but not limited to, therapists, therapy assistants, nurses, nursing home administrators, MDS coordinators and other professional staff.

Aedon Staffing is a large company that covers all 50 states, and can have you on assignment within one to two weeks. They offer personal service and are on a first name basis with their travelers. All of their travelers are able to get ahold of their recruiter after hours. They also have an after-hours answering service on their main number that can be contacted for any issues that may arise.

Benefits that they offer include: competitive pay, referral bonuses, direct deposit of paychecks, continuing education reimbursement, and a 401k SavingsPlus retirement plan. Their travel employees are also eligible for free first day medical insurance (single coverage), free first day dental insurance (single coverage), guaranteed pay, completion bonuses, travel reimbursement, free private housing, licensure and certification assistance, vision insurance, free accidental death and dismemberment insurance, free life insurance, and other voluntary benefit options.

Their parent company, Golden Ventures (aka Beverly Enterprises), has 380+ facilities nationwide that they staff. Their sister company, Aegis Therapies, staffs temporary employees through Aedon Staffing while they are looking for permanent hires. For more information you can contact them at 3816 W. Linebaugh Ave., Suite 301, Tampa, FL 33618, give them a call at 888-777-5305 or visit their website at www.aedonstaffing.com.

~*~

All Health Staffing

All Health Staffing offers Travel and Temp to Perm staffing jobs for Nurses, Therapists , Pharmacists and Operating Room/ Surgical Technicians throughout the United States , including Hawaii and Alaska . You can expect to be able to work within 2 weeks or less in most cases. The start time is dependent on several factors, including how quickly all paperwork is provided, completion of online testing, housing availability, etc.

All Health Staffing is a staffing agency that believes highly in character and commitment as much as they do in making a placement. Our foundation set firmly on principles of honesty, ethics and good moral fiber. You are treated with dignity and respect at all times and are not forgotten once the placement is made. They call the clinician often to make sure all is well. AHS believes service is extremely important, and it is the hallmark of their business. Many of their candidates come to them via referral; this would not happen if they didn't take care of the clinicians they already have with them.

All Health Staffing provides 24/7 support. If you need them after hours or on the weekend you can simply call their emergency number and you will speak with someone in short order who will be there to hear your concerns, and hopefully resolve the problem right away. They also provide a Nurse Practitioner as a consultant, and if there are any clinical issues that you have questions about, you can simply call to speak with their NP to get it resolved. They provide you with their emergency number for any type of emergencies, albeit for problems at work or with your apartment.

All Health Staff is considered a moderate-sized company that is big on service and pay. With their agency, travelers will be treated to individual attention to detail. You will receive an account representative who will be assigned to a particular traveler, and handle any service-related issues that may arise, which prevents the clinician from having to call housing, payroll, insurance, benefits, etc. It's all handled by the traveler's individual representative.

All Health Staffing offers a full array of benefits, such as free or furnished housing, low cost health insurance, relocation reimbursement, SIMPLE IRA retirement plan, 100% licensure reimbursement, uniform reimbursement and more. By law, all agencies have to carry a certain amount of professional liability insurance to protect them and the nurse if needed. They do provide adequate amounts of insurance. Specifically, they provide general and professional liability, as well as worker's compensation; however, the cost for the clinician to have self-insurance is relatively minor and they recommend that each person consider adding their own coverage, especially if they plan to job-hop between agencies often. As a rule, bonuses are taxed at a higher tax rate than normal salary. While some of their assignments do include a completion bonus, most of these are generated by the facility. They believe in paying you the highest possible salary they can, no matter the shift, no matter the day.

They are more than just another travel company because they provide top quality personal service to all of their clinicians, including calling them frequently during the assignment and resolving problems fairly and efficiently. It is their goal to empathize with their clients, and they view themselves as being in the clinician's predicament, so each time they aspire to treat their employees the way they would want to be treated.

They are very humble to have such great candidates, and while they thank God for their current and past clinicians, they thank God in advance for their future nurses too. Consider giving them a call, and remember, they will take care of the details. For more information, All Health Staffing can be found at 430 South 5th Street, Richmond, Texas 77469. Their toll free phone number is 877-577-8233. Their website is www.allhealthstaffing.com.

~*~

Alliant Medical Staffing

Alliant Medical Staffing offers both travel and permanent jobs for nurses and allied health professionals. The average time from acceptance of an application to the first day on the job is usually about two to three weeks, and they cover the entire United States. They are a small company. Unlike some of the larger travel staffing companies, a traveler is able to build a trusting relationship with their recruiter. The recruiter is their main point of contact for any issue, so the traveler always knows who to call and always has someone who can take action for them.

Alliant Medical Staffing goes out-of-the way to build personal relationships with all of their travelers. Their travelers don't have a different department to call for every type of problem. The recruiter acts as your single point-of-contact and coordinates with the appropriate departments to handle issues. They offer 24/7 support while their travelers are on assignment, so if there is ever a need for assistance they are only a phone call away.

Benefits that are available include a wide variety of assignment options, personal attention, higher wages, exceptional insurance coverage, free private housing, generous housing subsidies, sign-on bonuses, completion bonuses, loyalty bonuses, referral bonuses, tax-free travel allowances, reimbursements for continuing education, credentialing assistance, and license reimbursement.

Once you begin a relationship with Alliant Medical Staffing you will discover that what makes them different is that they give you personalized attention you deserve. Their recruiters take the time to understand your goals, preferences, and skills so they can match you to the assignment that best fits your needs.

Through unparalleled personal service their team consistently strives to make sure their travelers have nothing but the best experience possible. With Alliant Medical Staffing you can expect a wide variety of travel employment options, great compensation and benefits, fully furnished housing, and lucrative bonuses, not to mention a friendly voice on the other end of the phone if you ever need their assistance.

For more information you can contact them at 12655 N. Central Expressway, Suite 420, Dallas, TX 75243. They can be called at 866-868-0469 or visit them online at www.alliantmedcal.com.

~*~

American Traveler Staffing Professionals

American Traveler Staffing Professionals offer great assignments for travel nurses and physical therapists. Earn as much as $42/hour in such places as Charlottesville, VA, Columbia, SC, Washington, DC, Tucson, AZ, Greenville, NC, Beaumont, TX, Fairfield, CA, Newark, NJ, Springfield, VT, Georgetown, SC, and Richmond, VA. Great pay and bonuses are available. They can have you ready to go in about a week, and you will be treated as a person, not just a name.

You'll enjoy traveling to new destinations, working in fine teaching hospitals, living in glorious accommodations, and always earning great competitive salaries and compensation. Lucrative salaries, completion bonuses, double overtime, free group health, dental and life insurance, referral bonuses, licensure reimbursement, free weeks between assignments, loyalty bonuses, AAA membership, subsidy, CEU reimbursement, Protection Plus plan 401K, professional liability insurance, and workman's compensation.

As an American Traveler your consultant will be with you every step of the way. You'll experience the ultimate assignment because your consultant will find the one that meets your criteria for location, hospital specifications, housing, salary and bonuses. While you enjoy meeting new friends and living in exciting new places your consultant and the professional support staff at American Traveler will take care of all the important details like on-time paychecks, travel reimbursements, insurance, and benefits administration.

They can be found at 1615 S Federal Highway, Boca Raton, FL 33432. Their phone is listed as 800-884-8788. Their place on the web is located at www.americantraveler.com.

~*~

ATC Healthcare

ATC specializes in contract and per diem assignments for nursing and allied staff all over the United States. They are a medium-to-large company that is a publicly traded company without multi-layers of management and staff so "everybody knows you name." They can have you ready to go in one day to one week. From recruitment to client service, to housing and credentialing, ATC provides in-depth personal service to every healthcare professional they work with. If there are problems at nights, most recruiters provide their cell number, and there is always someone in the office from 7:00 a.m. to 9:00 p.m. and often on weekends.

Other benefits include medical insurance, dental insurance, 401k, sign-on and completion bonuses, direct deposit, free digital camera and cruise for consecutive assignment completions, housing and meal allowances paid weekly, not monthly. Also, there is adequate professional insurance.

They are more than just another staffing company, due to their vast experience in the healthcare field, one-on-one relationship-building service, contracts with hundreds of facilities across the country, and the ability to provide the best pay package in the industry. They can get you where you want to go and what you want to make. Just call them at 866-562-7667. They are located at 1983 Marcus Ave, Lake Success, NY 11042 or found on the web at www.atctravelers.com.

~*~

Attentive Healthcare

Attentive Healthcare has exciting opportunities nationwide for all healthcare professionals. They are working with some of the finest healthcare systems in the country, along with the rural hospitals. Attentive Healthcare can meet your needs with their divisions in traveling, per diem, or permanent placement.

Attentive Healthcare has been owned and operated by an RN traveler and a former RT/business owner since 1999, so they know the importance of a caring company. When they hire their staff, it is important that they treat their candidates with dignity and respect. Their whole goal is being able to connect with their healthcare professionals. Attentive Healthcare isn't about quotas;

it is about people. They currently have assignments throughout the United States, and they can have you ready to go in as little as one day to one month, depending on the facility and licensing. Your recruiter will keep you updated on the progress. Their recruiters and staff will always be upfront and honest with you. They work diligently to give you the assignments that best fit your desires and clinical skills. You are their #1 priority. Their Director of Recruitment, Sherri Wood, has been chosen three years in a row in the "Showcase of Recruiters of the Year." They are proud to have her representing Attentive Healthcare.

Being a "number" is not what they are all about. They know their travelers' names when they call and they want to know what is going on in their lives. Being an advocate for you is important to them. Attentive Healthcare has the feel of a "small company," but with all the "big company" benefits. Attentive Healthcare understands that everyone is different and has individual needs. They try to accommodate and be "attentive" to what their travelers' needs are. You can always reach a recruiter by phone, no matter what day or time you call. Their clinical representatives are available 24/7. They are always there for you.

Benefits include fully furnished private housing, direct deposit, healthcare benefits, travel reimbursements, completion bonuses on selected assignments, and top competitive pay. Attentive Healthcare gives each professional on assignment (free of change) a first dollar coverage (supplemental) medical policy with no deductibles, no pre-existing condition limitations and no co-insurance requirement. Attentive Healthcare covers 100% of the professional liability with one of the best companies in the nation.

They say, "Thank you for all you do as healthcare professionals. You make this world a better place. Attentive Healthcare would love the opportunity to give you a great experience. Join hands with us!"

For more information you can write to them at Attentive Healthcare, P.O. Box 6650, Sheridan, WY 82801. Phone calls can be made to 877-499-7606. Or you can visit their website at www.attentivehealthcare.net.

~*~

Bestaff Arcadia

Bestaff Arcadia has a high placement rate for emergency room, ICU, CCU, Med/Surg, trauma, step down, telemetry, correctional, psychiatric, and outpatient surgery. As part of the Arcadia Health Services group, they can also provide a broad range of non-travel opportunities between assignments, or for travelers wishing to take a break from travel. Finally, they are always interested in looking at qualified RNs to join their team in Kentucky. Currently, Bestaff has assignments in the majority of all of the United States, but they do not currently offer international assignments. A good estimate from confirmation to the first day of orientation would be 10 business days.

They are a medium-sized company with a special touch for treating every nurse with respect, courtesy and fairness. They are what their name says: a company that wants to provide a quality travel experience for their nurses. They are not looking to be the biggest or the fastest growing—just the best. In addition to having a personalized recruiter working to develop tailored packages/ assignments for each traveler, their Founder/Chief Nursing Officer is an RN who spends personal time working with their travelers to discuss issues (clinical and personal) related to their specific travel assignments.

Benefits provided include 401k, first-day insurance, private housing for every traveler, referral bonuses, and a loyalty/rewards recognition program. Their pay packages are among the highest in the industry.

Every individual in their company, from the president to the Chief Nursing Officer, from the recruiter to the receptionist answering the phone, knows that their job is to place nurses of the highest quality and make the travel assignments "hassle free" and a great experience for the traveler. According to many of their nurses, they provide the best housing and travel service, the best and most individualized contracts, the best ongoing field support, and the best pay-per-assignment. Most of their nurses return for several assignments. Their hospitals love their nurses and their nurses love their assignments. They really care about their nurses and enjoy taking care of even the smallest details.

For more information they can be found at 4223 Lexington Road, Paris, KY 40362. Their office number is listed as 866-988-2378 and they can be found online at www.bestaff.com.

~*~

Bridge Staffing Inc.

Bridge Staffing (BSI) offers travel contracts nationwide to travel professionals: RNs, LPNs, Techs. Most of the contract openings they receive are for 13 weeks. They also receive short term of four to eight weeks at times. They hold contracts in most of the 50 states. They also are able to receive job postings from Medifis in locations where they do not hold contracts. Most of the job postings they receive are on the average in 31-35 of the 50 states.

All of the BSI recruiters are home-based, which allows each of them to be more flexible in their working hours. When you are on the road it is very important to be able to reach your recruiter when you need to. All of the recruiters at BSI take the time to get to know their travelers. They want you to be comfortable with them.

Bridge Staffing ranks in the medium range. Their agency is based on "relationships." They take the time to get to know all of their travelers. They have a traveler ready to go in three to fourteen days. Many times this is in the hands of the facilities, based on needs and response times.

All BSI recruiters are based in their home offices. Each of their travelers has the numbers and email addresses to reach them. They have a 24-hour, toll free on-call. They have a secondary RN on-call for clinical issues. Their recruiters really care. They work with you individually to get as much as possible for you from each assignment. They provide honest answers to questions; they answer their phone and/or return calls.

Bridge Staffing is nurse owned and operated. Their benefits include a 1 bedroom, furnished, private apartment or a stipend, BCBS health and dental insurance with day 1 coverage (family coverage available—great rates!), $25,000.00 term life insurance, professional liability insurance, 401K, tax-free per diem, license and travel reimbursement, and 24-hour emergency clinical assistance. AFLAC group rates are now available. They also have loyalty incentives for long-term travelers. It is important that a company provides professional liability insurance to its employees. The coverage amounts will vary from one agency to another. The agency HR department should be able to provide you with coverage information. Your recruiter can also obtain this information for you. *Ask!*

What would they like travelers to know? "Always ask questions. There are many recruiters out there that are very good at sales. Make sure the deal is as good as it sounds. If you didn't understand something, ask again. Keep a notebook and write everything down."

Bridge Staffing is located at 3765B Government Blvd, Mobile, AL 36693 or can be phoned at 866-661-7070. Their website is located at www.bridgestaffing.com,

~*~

Cirrus Medical Staffing

Cirrus offers travel opportunities to nurses and allied health professionals. They also perform permanent placement of both nurses and allied health professionals, particularly in management and executive roles. You can expect a professionally fulfilling adventure, chocked full of lifetime experiences. They have contracts throughout all fifty states and work with hospitals of all sizes and flavors (for profit, not-for-profit, Indian Reservations, military, government, metropolitan, rural, etc.). They won't stand for their travelers being limited, so they encourage their travelers to try them all. The adventure of exerting flexibility in a small hospital to crisis-driven adventures of Level I trauma centers allows their travelers to become more seasoned professionals. Cirrus travelers develop the type of professional who has worked with various management styles and has the acquired talent to share with other facilities. The Cirrus adventure allows their travelers to remain true to their "calling," without losing touch with himself/herself or sacrificing career fulfillment.

Not only are they personal, they are as flexible as possible. They try to structure each contract according to their travelers' personal needs. This is why their retention rate has exceeded 70% during the last few years.

They are a medium-sized company, but still offer the same careful attention to detail with their travelers as when they were smaller. They know each of their traveler's names and contact them regularly. They're attentive to their travelers' issues and provide the backing for issues that may arise on assignments. They still correct their travelers' issues immediately. They have a 24-hour, 7 day a week emergency phone number that's answered by a Cirrus staff member, not an answering service.

Benefits include paid major medical, dental, vision, prescription discount program, life insurance (effective from day one), 401(k) with employer matching (2% of weekly income), PTO accrual, vacation pay, direct deposit, weekly pay, credit union, travel pay, tax advantage program, optional insurance such as financial planning, long-term care insurance, cancer insurance, accident insurance, STD, supplemental life insurance. You are also provided with paid liability insurance, paid private housing, utility stipends, license reimbursement, eight bonus programs, 24 x 7 emergency phone number, and permanent placement services. Cirrus is a Certified Healthcare Staffing Firm by the Joint Commission. The travelers' utilities are placed in Cirrus' name and they pay a monthly utility stipend that their travelers find comfortable and fair. Their professional liability insurance exceeds the standard limits that are required by healthcare facilities on their contracts. There is no need for the nurse to supply their own liability insurance whatsoever.

What makes them different is that they get to know their travelers personally, they correct any problems immediately, they support them when something goes wrong, and they recognize that there are two sides to each story. The hospitals aren't always "right." They reinvest heavily in their travelers. While other firms might be "buying" travelers, Cirrus prefers to offer a well-rounded package with premium insurance coverage and policies that create security for their travelers *and* pay them well. In other words,

Cirrus is concerned with providing a comprehensive compensation package that is above industry standards for their travelers.

They regard each traveler's requests seriously and try to always do what's right to create a win/win situation; however, they can't be everything to everybody. What you can depend on is that they *do* win your trust and don't violate it. They're truthful in their communications and they do what's right for their travelers.

Cirrus contractually ensures that your hours are guaranteed through the facility to which you are assigned. Furthermore, if you're sick or have an emergency, not only will you be supported by your Cirrus recruiter, but you will be allowed to make up your lost time.

Cirrus treats each traveler with respect, and they form lasting relationships based on honesty and doing what they say they'll do. They pride themselves in finding the right assignment for your needs.

Cirrus Medical Staffing is different in the fact that they give their travelers the individual attention and flexibility they need in order to perform their jobs successfully. They go the extra mile to ensure that their travelers are safely housed, supported with their issues, and treated with the respect they deserve. Their travelers are treated as the professionals they are and served as the company's most important asset (because they are). Cirrus is known in the travel community for being fair, doing what they say they will do, and for doing what is right. Some of their most experienced travelers can attest to how well they are treated and how quickly they respond to traveler issues/concerns. Their response and resolution time is commended by their travelers and their yearly traveler satisfaction survey has been sterling since their inception.

For more information, you can contact Cirrus Medical Staffing, 4651 Charlotte Park Drive, Suite 400, Charlotte, NC 28217. You can call them at 1-800-299-8132, fax them at 800-506-5309, email them at travel@cirrusmedicalstaffing.com or visit their website at www.cirrusmedicalstaffing.com.

~*~

Client Solv Healthcare

Client Solv offers 13-week travel contracts, permanent placement, and long-term contracts, all at no cost to the RN, with placement in all 50 states available. They have no international assignments at this time. Application to an assignment time is about two-to-four weeks, depending on the facility & RN needs.

Personal service is an absolute! Recruiters are available to personally serve each traveler's needs, and they have an on-call representative 24/7.

About professional insurance—do you believe that the insurance that a company provides is good enough, or does the nurse also need to obtain her own professional insurance?

They are a small company, but growing. However, they plan to limit their growth in order to maintain the personal relationships they currently enjoy with their RNs. All of their RN's are treated with the utmost respect and sense of urgency.

Client Solv Health Care's benefits include a minimum pay rate of $30.00/hr. This is guaranteed, and it is included in their web site. Although they do not match employee's contribution into their 401k Plan, they can participate immediately. Their travel reimbursement is flat rate ($500.00 round trip) for a 13-week contract. The travel is payable once again if the nurse extends their contract. It would be pro-rated if the extension is less than 13 weeks.

In addition to the free private housing option, they also offer a minimum of $1,200.00 a month in housing allowance should the nurse prefer that option. Utilities are capped at $100.00 a month, with the nurse paying any difference via a payroll deduction. It is very rare that this happens.

CEU reimbursement is capped at $500.00 per year. It includes ACLS, PALS, and NRP recertification. If a nurse wants a completion bonus, that can be offered, but frankly they prefer to take that money and put it into their salary. They do offer sign-on bonuses for select assignments, payable with the nurse's first full paycheck. Direct deposit is available every other week. Per policy, they offer a minimum of one (1) sick day per 13-week contract without financial penalty, but depending on extenuating circumstances, they have provided more days. Professional liability insurance is also offered to the nurse. They also pay $500.00 to a nurse who refers someone to their company for employment. The referral bonus is paid when the referred person has completed their first full pay period.

They approach their assignments in a very different way from the other companies out there. They don't try to push an RN into the jobs they already have; they find out where he/she wants to go, and they market him/her specifically to those facilities. In fact, they market directly to the hiring managers! The benefit here is that only one profile is submitted, so the nurse manager is able to screen the file and open the order with them. This ensures that the RN is getting only the assignments he/she is looking for.

Their philosophy is that a happy traveler is a loyal traveler, so they do what very few other agencies do: they listen! By doing so, they have put together a package that gives travelers everything they have been searching for in a Travel Nursing Company, and RNs get this great package without having to sacrifice anything! Amazing concept, eh? If the RN would prefer to trade in some of his/her benefits for a higher hourly salary, they can certainly do that.

For more information, Client Solv can be found at 7730 E. Belleview Ave, Suite A201, Englewood, CO 80111. They are just a phone call away also at 888-500-7658. Their website is located at www.clientsolvhealthcare.com.

~*~

Comforce Travel Nurses Unlimited

Comforce TNU offers travel assignments for nurses and allied health professionals, with opportunities in all areas except psychiatric and rehab. They also have temp-to-hire positions for RNs and LVNs. They mainly offer assignments in California, but occasionally they have assignments in other states. They are constantly adding more facilities, so nurses should always check in with them to see what is new.

Their recruiters are always available and they look out for the traveler's best interest. They try to meet each nurse's individual needs by providing different packages on each assignment. A travel nurse can expect to have contact with one recruiter throughout her employment. They also have a person there who helps with credentialing and housing that a nurse may hear from every now and again.

Comforce is a large company, but the travel nursing division is very small, with a total of four nursing recruiters. They have a director of medical staffing who has been an on-sight manager at a hospital who holds all of their recruiters to a very high ethical standard. You can be sure that you will be treated as a name and not a number.

Since they are the vendor managers at most of the hospitals they work with, they usually get a 24-48 hr. turn-around between submittal of initial paperwork of application acceptance, reference checks, and the first phone interview. After that it depends on how quickly the applicant can get the other things done, such as a physical, TB test, Skills and HIPPA tests, license and CPR renewal etc., so it can take a few days or it can take a few weeks.

They have an on-site office at most of the hospitals they work with, so if there is a problem a nurse can speak to someone from Comforce right away. They have someone 24/7 to answer your questions.

They offer high-paying assignments, free fully furnished apartments or stipend, relocation, rental car, insurance, 401K, and a great referral program. Their referral program offers nurses the ability to make up to $5,000 just for referring their friends. They offer loyalty bonuses on each assignment completed after the first assignment. Also, they have an employee discount club, which is good for tourist attractions, movies, etc., and they have someone available 24/7 for problems. They also have RNs on their staff to help with any clinical problems. They also have weekly pay with direct deposit. They offer free malpractice insurance while on assignment, which should be enough, but there is no harm in a nurse getting their own too.

Comforce is unique in many ways. They have on-site offices at most of their hospitals so there is always someone a nurse can physically go to if there is a problem. Comforce works with prestigious hospitals and always makes sure that the hospitals have a safe environment. They have over 40 years of experience in the staffing industry, so they know what works. They are here to make your travel assignment hassle-free.

The travel nursing division at Comforce is small, which means that they can offer the travelers the personal attention they need. Comforce is the vendor/manager at several hospitals, which means that even other travel companies will have to go through a Comforce employee to get their nurses submitted for an assignment.

Comforce has been in the staffing industry for over 40 years, so nurses can expect a solid foundation. They are constantly growing, too, so nurses should always stay in touch to see what new positions they have.

Comforce Travel Nurses Unlimited is located at 17682 Mitchell North, Suite 100, Irvine, CA 92614. They can be contacted by phone at 800-660-9544. Their company website can be found at www.comforcetravelrn.com.

~*~

Cross Country Staffing

Cross Country Staffing has placement services for travel and per diem RNs, LPNs, Certified Surgical Technologists, Respiratory Care Practitioners, PTAs, OTAs, Imaging Professionals, Pharmacists, Medical Laboratory Professionals, Registered PT, OT and SLP Professionals. They are unique in that they work with just about every hospital that takes traveling nurses. They find out where the travel nurse wants to go and they make every effort to place them there. During national disasters they are also one of the top providers of nurses to the disaster regions. Related to the fact that they do a lot of vender management in which they personally do the interviews, your assignment can be confirmed within 24 hours.

They are very customer-service oriented, and the fact that their company has grown so large is related to the fact that most of their nurses are from referrals. Once the nurse refers another nurse to their recruiter, that recruiter helps the referred nurse obtain an assignment in their area of choice. If the nurse-to-recruiter personality isn't a perfect fit, they make every attempt to make sure that the nurse's needs are met.

They not only cover all of the United States, but also the US Virgin Islands and Bermuda. Through their partner, Assignment America, they offer assignments in the United States to candidates from Canada, the United Kingdom, Australia, South America, Ireland, New Zealand, Trinidad and Jamaica.

Cross Country is a very large company and every effort is made for their nurses not to get lost in the system. They pride themselves on top-rated customer service. They have a quality control team that makes sure that the hospital is supplied with only the best nurses and that the nurses work with only the top-notched recruiters. They have a 24-hour phone number for all their nurses so they can reach a manager on call. They have nurse managers who will assist the nurses with any clinical questions or situations that develop.

Benefits depend on your specialty, experience and assignment location. They always negotiate top rates for their travelers. Add in shift differentials and completion bonuses of up to $3,500 and you'll see why Cross Country leads the industry in total compensation-pay and benefits. They offer completion bonuses on many assignments. You can earn from $500 to $3500 on certain assignments. They also guarantee your hours. You will be paid for low census shifts in excess of 24 hours, which cannot be made up during the assignment on a guaranteed pay assignment. They have thousands of guaranteed pay assignments throughout the United States in a variety of settings and specialties. With their referral bonus program you can receive $500 for every healthcare professional you refer to Cross Country who begins their first travel assignment or accepts a permanent position. Their comprehensive salary and benefits package includes completion and referral bonuses, shift differentials, a 401(k) retirement plan, free first day health, dental and life insurance, free housing or a generous housing allowance free first-day professional liability, short-term disability insurance and accidental death coverage, travel reimbursement, free checking and direct deposit, continuing education, and discounts on products and services at some of the nation's top retailers. All standard benefits begin as soon as you start your assignment. Each nurse that travels with them will have their own personal professional insurance. Even if the nurse only works for 13 weeks, their coverage lasts for the full year.

They constantly listen to input and ideas from their nurses. They provide many services, including educational opportunities, testing programs, and a lot of their recruiters are nurses and have been out there on the road themselves. They also provide in-house corporate counsel.

Do your homework and look at the total package. They provide a lot more soft items than any other travel company out there. Their nurses and allied health employees don't have to worry about whether or not they are going to be in compliance with the IRS at the end of the year, because they follow the strict guidelines and have a professional staff that keeps track of any changes. They also would like to dispel the rumor that all of their nurses have shared housing, when in fact only about 15% have shared housing, and your housing, along with other amenities, gets better and better through their Loyalty Rewards program.

For more information you can find them at 6552 Park of Commerce Blvd., Boca Raton, FL 33487. They are also available by phone at 800-530-6125. They can be found online at www.cctc.com.

~*~

Curastat

Curastat has contract, direct hire, travel, and per diem opportunities available on the east and west coasts and between, but they do not cover the entire U.S. As with many companies, they are continuously expanding into new markets and rely heavily on their current employees' desired locations in where they put their efforts. Their average is around three weeks, although they have experienced much quicker and much longer time frames.

They are a small-to-medium-sized company and everyone can expect to be treated as a person. The growth that they have experienced has been directly related to their current employees' referrals. Although their employees benefit financially from their referrals, their newly-referred employees have said that their decisions have been based on the positive experiences the Curastat employees have shared with them. They appreciate their employee base and want to give them a reason to stay with them.

Benefits include weekly direct deposit, certification renewals after six months of continuous employment, referral bonuses, and licensure reimbursement.

A great reputation is very important to Curastat. They want to provide as much information to both their employees and their clients as possible. Obviously, it is important for them to make placements. It is even more important for them to make every effort to ensure that the placement is a success; i.e. a good match. They are happy to answer any additional questions a travel nurse may have.

For more information, you can contact them at 2141 E. Camelback Rd., Suite 250, Phoenix, AZ 85016 or reach them by phone at 888-865-7828. They can be found on the web at www.curastat.com.

~*~

Dakota Med Temps

Dakota Med Temps (DMT) has both long and short-term assignments for RNs and LPNs nationwide. They have private and government contracts so they are able to place nurses almost anywhere. They have assignments throughout the United States, including Alaska and Hawaii. Typically, you can be on location in two or three weeks, depending on the facility the nurse would like to work in.

As a small staffing company they really get to know their nurses and take care of them. Their recruiters are nurses themselves and understand the demands of the profession in a travel setting or a permanent placement. They do all they can to accommodate their nurses and find the best fit for them and the facilities they work with. A majority of their nurses stay with Dakota Med Temps, Inc. for at least two 13-week contracts, many for more because of the way they are treated by the DMT staff.

DMT is a very small company. All of their nurses are treated with respect and are called by name. Even their receptionist is able to recognize many nurses by the sound of their voice when they call! Their nurse recruiters have cell phones and they give that number out at their discretion. If a nurse cannot get ahold of their recruiter overnight their issue will be addressed first thing in the morning.

Travel, housing, per diem, medical, vision and dental coverage, supplemental insurance, simple IRA, flex-spending account, referral bonuses, retention bonus, license reimbursement are just a few of they benefits offered. All DMT nurses are required to provide their own professional liability insurance coverage in addition to the company plan.

Their recruiters care about their nurses and work hard to make sure they are comfortable and happy with their assignments. DMT offers comparable benefits to most other travel companies, but offers the personal touch to their nurses.

Dakota Med Temps can be found at 201 Pine Ave, Hill City, SD 57745. Their phone number is 605-574-9024. They can be found online at www.dakotamedtemps.com.

~*~

Expedient Medstaff

Expedient is a small company with a mission to be known as "the easiest company to do business with." Travelers can fully expect to be treated by name with VIP services. They have assignments in nearly every state and can have travelers processed in as quickly as one day. They operate very comfortably with a two-to-seven-day window. They have a team that is assigned specifically to their travelers and each member is an expert in their aspect of the travel business. Their travelers can expect the best from assignment to return home and beyond.

They have someone available at all times, including a nurse advocate team to solve clinical or hospital issues. This team is comprised of registered nurses; each member has over twelve years of nursing experience.

Benefits offered currently include Blue Cross Blue Shield PPO with vision, dental, chiropractic, and prescription coverage. Their health benefits are available from day one. Also available are the following insurances: disability, hospitalization, cancer, personal accident, specified health event, and they even offer insurance for their travelers' pets. They also have a 401k to shelter income for retirement.

Expedient is different from other companies in that their senior management team has over forty years experience in healthcare staffing. Secondly, they have a Nurse Advocate Team that makes sure their traveler assignments are personally and professionally rewarding and clinically safe. They also have a Travel Tax Guarantee. They guarantee that, based on the information provided by their travelers, their pay packages will be compliant with the IRS rules and regulations. Thirdly, their Housing Manager has a business degree in logistics and holds a professional real estate license. This expertise can be counted on for those travelers needing housing.

Expedient treats their travelers like a client. They value their travelers and treat them with respect and gratitude. They know their travelers have other options. With every interaction they try to remind their travelers that they made the right choice when nurses chose them.

They can be reached at Expedient Medstaff, One Heritage Place, Suite 250, Southgate, MI 48195 or phone them at 877-367-8770. Their website can be found at: www.expedientmedstaff.com

~*~

Fastaff

Fastaff is one of the top 5 national travel nursing companies. Since 1989 FASTAFF has been a leading healthcare staffing company. Their nurses earn top pay, receive exceptional benefits, bonuses and fully paid travel/housing.

They offer travel assignments in some of the most prestigious facilities in the nation. With assignments ranging from 8-13 weeks and guaranteed hours, FASTAFF strives to give their travel nurses the opportunity to work where they want to and when they want to while still maintaining the lifestyle they desire. Normally, from the time that your file is complete until the first day on the job is an average of seven to ten days, but with Fastaff, nurses go to work immediately.

Fastaff benefits include pay rates up to $48 per hour, loyalty bonus up to $10,000 per year, flexible benefits starting on day one, assignments starting at 8 weeks with guaranteed hours, fully paid travel and quality housing, perks program for discounts on products and services including Dell, AAA and more. Friendship has its rewards; refer a nurse and earn up to $3,000, comprehensive!

Because Fastaff values its nursing professionals, they give you the assignments you want with the benefits you deserve. When you join their team, you know you'll be working for top pay at some of the finest healthcare facilities in the country. FASTAFF strives to find work that is professionally fulfilling and personally rewarding.

To find out more check them out at www.fastaff.com. They can be found at 6501 S. Fiddler's Green Circle, Suite 200, Greenwood Village, CO 80111 or reached be phone at 888-890-1924.

~*~

Freedom Healthcare

Freedom Healthcare Staffing (FreedomHCS) offers temporary travel assignments from four to thirteen weeks in duration all over the United States. Typically, a response from the hospital is within two to three business days; some hospitals are quicker with a response and some are slower. The important thing, for them, is to advise the Healthcare traveler on their experience on working with a particular hospital and to set realistic expectations for the turnaround time on an interview and ultimately an offer of a position.

One of their core values is to treat their Healthcare travelers with respect. Although they are a small company, Freedom Healthcare Staffing was established by executives from the hospital and staffing industry. Many of their nurses know them from the larger companies they were formally with. It is very important to their president, as well as every member of Freedom Healthcare staffing, that their Healthcare travelers have a rewarding experience, both intrinsically and monetarily, while working with their company.

All of their staff is on call 24 hours a day, including their President! You can be assured that if you do have a problem you will not be routed to a call center, but to an individual within FreedomHCS that is empowered to handle your particular situation.

They offer comprehensive benefit insurance thru United Healthcare, life insurance, Simple IRA with Company match, CEU reimbursement, licensing assistance, professional liability insurance, direct deposit, weekly pay, online portal, company-provided housing and travel, along with a lucrative referral rewards program.

Freedom Healthcare Staffing stands behind their Healthcare Travelers! Many companies pay "lip service" to this value, but this is also at the heart of their interaction with their nurses. In fact, there are hospital clients they will no longer do business with due to their perceived treatment of their Healthcare travelers.

It is their goal to make every experience with Freedom Healthcare Staffing rewarding. They also specialize in the "hand-holding" sometimes needed for first-time travelers, and for that matter, anyone else who needs some extra emotional support while on the road. Please visit them at www.freedomhcs.com or give them a call at 866-463-0385. They can be found at: 2600 S. Parker Road, Suite 6-360, Denver, CO 80014.

~*~

Gemini Med Staffing

Gemini Med Staffing offers permanent and temporary staffing. They can do assignments from a per diem status to six month contracts. For permanent recruitment they find the position you desire in the area you prefer. They can handle all the negotiations with the hiring facility to make your relocation comfortable, in which all fees are paid by the facility. Currently they staff the United States proper and the US Virgin Islands.

Nurses move pretty quickly upon application. They have tried to make their hire-on process simple to assist the nurses in obtaining assignments in a timely manner. They treat all their travelers as friends. They are small and began as an allied health care agency. They are very excited that they are venturing into nursing.

They hope each professional listed obtains the assignment they want with the benefits they desire. Each is treated with respect as they understand the challenges faced as a traveler. They have a recruiter on call twenty-four hours a day, seven days a week, three hundred and sixty-five days a year.

Although they are sometimes temporary, the benefits may include or be limited to private corporate housing or tax free lodging allowance, free utilities, free basic cable, pre-paid airfare or mileage, rental car or tax free transportation allowance, daily tax free meal allowance, tax free medical insurance, stipend, weekly direct deposit, worker's compensation and professional liability. Everyone at GMS is committed to serving you with top pay, medical insurance reimbursement, tax free meal allowances, pre-paid travel, rental car and private lodging OR travel, transportation and lodging allowances. You choose! With over two decades of national staffing experience, they know that they can provide world class customer service. Contact a recruiter today to secure your job in the nursing industry, let GMS make it as easy as you deserve it to be!

About professional insurance, there are two thoughts 1) It is good enough, however if an agency and an employee are in a situation, remember who is actually accused of the problem, the provider (nurse) or the agency. You should always protect yourself.

2) If you carry the extra insurance could it open you up for a situation? (My opinion: I would carry it but not talk too loudly about it.)

With nearly 30 years combined healthcare recruitment experience, their owners understand the staffing process and have determined that each employee in the "field" is the foundation for the business. If the travelers are not treated well the business will not survive. They work for their employees, and they are grateful they will choose to share their time on the road with them.

They say they would love for those who know them to spread the word about them and those who don't to give them a try! They are in the process of updating their website to include more nursing information and checklists. Check them out at 11672 E. Manzanita Trail, Dewey, AZ 86327. You can give them a call at 866-296-8164 or visit their website at www.geminimedstaff.com

~*~

Guardian Healthcare Staffing Solutions

Guardian Healthcare is a small company that prides itself on always trying to make it better for the nurse. Their nurses deserve the best and they are here to serve their nurses. From the time of application they can have you ready to go in one to three weeks on the average, and they provide assignments all over the United States. They offer professional travel assignments and permanent placement opportunities for both RN's and LPN's that are well matched for the nurse and the facility across the United States.

They offer full benefits which include full insurance coverage including, Blue Cross Blue Shield medical, dental and vision. They also offer sick day allowance for each assignment, $1,000 plus referral bonuses, $300 consecutive assignment referral bonuses, completion bonuses, loyalty awards, private housing accommodations, free utilities up to $100 per month and much more...

The owners decided to start their own Healthcare Staffing Company for one reason: they can and will always do what is the best for the nurse. Guardian Healthcare Staffing Solutions would love a chance to gain and keep your business. They are here to serve and provide solutions for you.

For More Information Contact: Guardian Healthcare Staffing Solutions, 4302 Live Oak Circle, Florence, SC 29501 or give them a call at: 800-670-7640. They can be found online: www.guardianhss.com.

~*~

Healthcare Professional Staffing

Healthcare Professional Staffing (HPS) specializes in allied professionals, physical, occupational, speech and respiratory therapists and clinical professionals, dialysis nurses, L&D nurses, ER nurses and cath lab nurses. HPS's staff consists of registered nurses and therapists who are now recruiters and marketing representatives. Their clients are in the USA. They do business in Alaska and Hawaii as well, but the majority of their work is in the continental USA. They can have you ready to go in three to five days, or however long it takes to get a state license.

Personal service and an incredible attention to detail is what they pledge to their employees. Here is an email from one of their employees. "Thank you so much for the gift basket. I got all kinds of goodies. You guys are wonderful and thoughtful. Truly, Wanda."

They are a small company and treat their employees as part of the HPS family. They have a 24 hour on-call phone where their employees can reach them.

Benefits at HPS include tuition reimbursement, free CEU's, legal support and psychological counseling. Their professional liability insurance is top-of-the-line and only costs the employee $28.66/month. Benefits include major medical, dental, vision, long and short-term disability, prescription drug plan and a life insurance policy.

Their internal staff is the key that makes them different. They truly care about their nurses and therapists. They exchange pictures of their children, share stories, and get involved with their staff. They have a 96% retention rate with their staff members. Call Healthcare Professional Staffing and experience the difference. Adventure, travel and great pay rates at 800-706-5493 or drop by and visit them at 7000 Central Parkway, Atlanta, GA 30328. Their website is located at www.hpsstaffing.com.

~*~

Healthcare Seeker

Healthcare Seeker offers travel positions for both nursing and allied professionals all over the United States. Personal service is one of the top reasons their travelers stay on with them. When you are a traveler with them, you stay with the recruiter you initially sign on with.

They are a medium-sized, family-owned company. You will definitely be treated as an individual, and definitely not a number. The average time from application to ready-to-go would be one to two weeks; although they have had some instances of a 48-hour turn-around time!

Though they cannot stress enough how personal their service is and how well they work with the individual needs of a traveler, they do offer free fully-furnished private housing, travel reimbursement, day-one medical coverage, free direct deposit that starts for your first paycheck, and much more. They have top-notch professional and liability insurance, but they feel it is a good idea for a travel nurse to obtain her own as well.

They treat their travelers the way they'd want to be treated—with respect! They find them housing they'd be willing to stay in themselves and pay them more than the rest of the industry.

For more information, they can be found at 612 Main Street, Boonton, NJ 07005 or can be phoned at 888-331-3431. Their website is located at www.healthcareseeker.com

~*~

Health Force

Health Force is a company that supplies RN and Allied Health travel assignments from Maine to Alaska. They try to assist you in obtaining the travel career that best suits your needs. They offer travel assignments for both Allied and nursing in most states. Typically, the assignments are 8-13 weeks in length. Occasionally, they also have shorter terms available. They take pride in the quality of health care they help to deliver. Finally, their seasoned, experienced staff is able to deliver a very caring and hands-on approach to their travelers. They cover as much of the US as they can. They are always calling new areas and hospitals to see where they can help. Every month they add new clients to their database.

They are a small-to-medium sized agency by design so they can give that personal touch. Their recruiters don't handle hundreds of travelers, and most of their in-house employees know the names of all of their field reps. Personal service is their main focus. They choose to remain a small-to-medium sized agency so this can be accomplished. They are a true partner for the traveler and hospital. Their sales team will market to an area where you want to go. They cater to special needs and make your package according to what you need, not to what they think you need.

They have someone on call 24 hours a day, 7 days a week for both housing and hospital issues. They promise a 2-hr. callback time. If you leave a message for the recruiter on call someone will try to help you. They also have an after-hours housing line. They do have an after-hours emergency line that you can contact if you have a situation that needs immediate attention. Their recruiter on call and housing on call have a 2-hr. callback window for those extreme issues, otherwise they recommend for situations that are not as serious to contact your recruiter or their manager first thing in the morning, during regular business hours.

Health Force provides a comprehensive benefits package, including complete health care coverage. They pay on time, every time, and are a true partner with you while you are in the field. In addition, the variety of assignments they are able to offer can get you to your desired location, with the pay and assignment length you're looking for. They have Anthem Blue Cross/Blue Shield health and dental insurance at a small cost to you and a portion of your premiums are paid by Health Force. They also provide free private housing with all assignments, and rental car/airfare with most. They have a referral program and tax advantage program to help you make more money on your travels. They are always looking to make their business better, so hopefully in the future there will be more benefits to talk about. They feel that they protect their fellow employees to the fullest with the professional insurance coverage they provide. They have heavily invested in insurance, but the bottom line is that each traveler needs to self-educate themselves and decide if it is necessary to carry their own professional insurance. They would never discourage a professional from obtaining personal protection, but they do carry a substantial professional policy with the traveler in mind.

Average turnaround time varies according to available assignments, the qualifications of the traveler and the documentation that they have readily available. This is a hard question. If your file is complete and they have a compatible job, most of their clients are ready to move and accept a profile within 48 hours. There are so many variables that go into a placement; the average placement could take 48 hrs. to 2 weeks. They push their clients for 2-3 day turnarounds for the best interest of everyone.

Health Force has worked for "the other" travel companies—the larger, less personal ones—been there before. They are not trying to recreate the largest business in town. They want to build a company of people that know and trust each other, relationships that last on both the employee and client side; all of these partnerships are important. They are made up of people with deep experience in the travel-staffing marketplace. They come from one of the largest agencies in the business, yet they decided to build Health Force very differently, with an uncompromised focus on the needs of each and every traveler. It is their people that makes them unique. They make a difference in the lives of travelers every day. Talk to their travelers, visit their site and see what they have to say, and you will see the Health Force difference firsthand when you travel with them.

For more information contact them at 10921 Reed Hartman Highway, Cincinnati, OH 45242 or give them a call at 800-811-6642. Their website is located at www.health-force.com

~*~

Health Providers Choice

Health Providers Choice (HPC) is seeking Registered Nurses/ Healthcare professionals. They are looking for personal, professional, and financial growth. You will find that they strive to be an employer of choice within the healthcare network market. HPC offers the seasoned professional many ways to achieve their professional goals of (1) Per-Diem: Work on a short-term basis; assignments range from one day to several weeks; (2) Contract: Guaranteed assignments for terms of 8-26 weeks within Michigan healthcare facilities; (3) Travel: Travel assignments throughout the United States. Their travelers enjoy the best benefits in the industry.

Health Providers Choice has five offices in Michigan, two offices in Arizona, and a Canadian Office in Windsor, Ont. to offer their nurse's employment opportunities throughout the United States and over international borders. They are committed to placing professionals that meet the stringent demands of healthcare needs in a timely matter. They employ only highly skilled and qualified healthcare professionals. They insure the quality of each selected candidate through a results-based behavioral interview and an in-depth screening and criteria review. Ninety-four percent (94%) of their nurses, upon completion of the hiring requirements for HPC, should expect to be placed immediately. They are committed to being accessible, responsive, and accountable to their nurses, clients, the staffing personnel, facility staff, and the patients they care for.

HPC has a small-company philosophy with a large presence nationwide that offers dedication, commitment, and that personal touch every nurse is looking for. Their mission, which they strive to achieve on a daily basis, is not just about putting a practitioner to work; it is about working for the practitioner. They have implemented an enhanced employee assistance and work/life program because they understand that because of today's stressful lifestyles it is harder than ever to balance work and family life. This program offers 24/7 toll-free access to trained and licensed professionals who are there to help with counseling with personal issues, child and elder care research and referrals, legal information, financial consultation, critical incident support, and online personal health information. As an alliance of Health Partners Incorporated and HP Personnel, HPC has more than 27 years of maturity and experience in serving the healthcare community. The HP Corporation has placed over 5,000 professionals in temporary, temp-to-hire, and permanent positions. Health Providers Choice understands that their professionals work around the clock. In order to service those who have different schedules than their office they have a 24-hour on-call support telephone line that is available to their nurses 7 days a week.

At Health Providers Choice they recognize the value of their professionals. Because of this, they have implemented a number of unique benefits, including highly competitive pay rates, complete shift flexibility with no minimum commitment, immediate-upon-hire health care coverage including medical, dental, vision, life insurance, short-term disability, 401K plan, weekly plan with direct deposit, referral bonuses, free continuing education, 24-hour administrative nursing support, vacation accrual based on time worked, license reimbursement, credential reimbursement, travel expenses, furnished housing, paid utilities for travel contracts, $250 tuition reimbursement after one full year of employment and both professional liability insurance and workman's compensation

All agencies are not the same. HPC is founded on the principle that healthcare professionals are, and always will be, independent practitioners with extreme value to each life they encounter and the hospital systems they support. Many of the professionals that are currently employed at Health Providers Choice describe their employment experience with HPC as "empowering." The same weary, underpaid, stressed, often angry and disenchanted professionals, searching for an alternative to their current job, can find empowerment by working with HPC—working their way, at their pace, and in their style. Ninety percent (90%) of their professionals come to them by referral, proving that they truly do stand behind their nurses and their commitment to them.

If a nurse is looking for a premiere staffing company with state-of-the-art standards of practice, a high-touch approach to recruiting, and a dynamic vision for the future of healthcare in America, you will be happy you joined the Health Providers Choice team.

For more information contact 691 N. Squirrel Road, Auburn Hills, MI 48326. They can be phoned at 888-299-9800. Their website can be found at www.hpcnursing.com.

~*~

Hospital Support

Hospital Support offers many assignments across the United States, except for Hawaii, and the time from application to the time you are on assignment usually depends on the facility. They pride themselves in personal service and the fact that the RNs deal specifically with the owners.

Hospital Support is a small company in which you can expect to be treated as a partner, with someone available to answer your questions twenty-four hours a day, seven days per week.

As a Hospital Support employee (non-independent contractor), they'll pay you the maximum hourly affordable rate, with double-time for over-time (with most contracts), absolutely free private housing or a non-taxed weekly or monthly housing subsidy paid directly to you. They will pay you $500-$1000 completion bonus, based on the contract. If the facility pays a completion bonus, you will receive all of it. You'll get free health insurance of up to $150/month, or they will give you $150/month towards your own coverage, travel reimbursement based on what you need to get there, tax advantage where you would not pay taxes on $14.65 of your hourly rate, also called per diem. They have 401K participation with matching, licensure reimbursement, weekly pay, direct deposit and more. As an employee, the company professional insurance should be enough that you don't necessarily have to purchase additional insurance.

Hospital Support is a temporary healthcare staffing company based in Austin, Texas. Hospital Support is a small company with a low overhead. They do not do much advertising because it's expensive and they would rather put more money in their nurse's pockets. They do not spend much money on flashy prints because again, it's expensive and they'd rather pay their nurses more. They get most of their candidates by referral; therefore, if you know any RNs, please tell them about Hospital Support.

For more information about Hospital Support you can write to them at the following address: 7801 North Lamar Blvd. Suite B-161, Austin, TX 78752, or phone them at 1-888-451-9996. Their website is located at www.HospitalSupport.com.

~*~

HRN Services

HRN provides travel opportunities for RNs throughout the country, as well as local per diem opportunities in areas in which they have local offices. HRN serves 47 of the 50 states. They do not offer international assignments at this time.

At HRN, the nurse signs their paychecks, which means that each employee of HRN recognizes that without the nurse, none of them would have a job! HRN travel coordinators walk the nurse through the paperwork process; then the nurse is asked about submissions prior to being submitted to any facility. The nurse is involved and approves all housing decisions prior to leases being signed. Their job is to facilitate the contract for the nurse and make it as seamless as possible, yet allowing the nurse to be a part of the decision-making process. They are a medium-to-large company. Their nurses are their business, never just a number. An HRN/RN director is on call after hours to assist with any issues that may arise.

They offer company-paid medical/dental benefits that are considered the best in this industry; also included are 401K, life insurance and work bonuses, superior company-paid housing, travel stipends and excellent pay. HRN provides malpractice insurance for their employees. They are divided on the issue of whether or not a nurse needs to supplement that insurance, as they have seen attorneys go after the nurse once they find out that there is more money available when involved in litigation. What HRN provides is adequate and has covered every nurse who has been involved in litigation.

HRN has collectively over 35 years experience in this industry. Many directors in the company are former travel nurses themselves, so they understand issues that are important to the nurse, and they make those a priority. The CEO of HRN is serious when he says that the nurse signs their paycheck and every employee of HRN realizes this concept. HRN is a company that stands behind their nurses. They are your advocate and they go the extra mile to take care of their nurses.

For more information they can be contacted at 8383 Wilshire Blvd, Suite 258, Beverly Hills, CA 90211, or give them a call at 800-476-5561. Their website can be found at www.hrnservices.com.

~*~

Intelistaf

InteliStaf Travel, a Division of Medical Staffing Network, takes care of their nurses and allied professionals. They meet their individual needs and accommodate their unique situations. They have travel and per diem available nationwide. Their main goal is very personal service to the RN who is representing InteliStaf. They can have you ready to go in a minimum of two weeks—sometimes less than two weeks, depending on the hospital requirements.

They are a large company with personal service; you will never be just a number to InteliStaf. They always have a recruiter on call 24/7.

Benefits include iRewards, paid time-off, referral bonus incentives, health, dental, vision, short-term disability, and life insurance. Also included are license reimbursement and certification reimbursement (ACLS, TNCC, ENPC, CCRN, but not BLS). They have free private housing with paid utilities except for phone and cable. They also use corporate housing that has everything, including weekly maid service in most medium-to-larger cities. Payroll is weekly for most clients; travel money, 401K with matching monies is also available. Their professional insurance is absolutely good enough to cover any travel or per diem RN.

They have many long-term travelers. The lead recruiter has been there for eleven years and has many RNs that have been with her that whole time and others that still keep in touch with them over the years that refer RNs to them. They are very honest and upfront about contracts, hospitals, benefits, etc. They never mislead their RNs in any way, shape or form.

InteliStaf is a large travel nurse company with more personalized service than any other large travel company. They are also one of the first travel companies, established in 1980. InteliStaf's goal is to hire qualified RNs and Allied Professionals that will provide high-quality care to patients.

For more RN information you can contact them at 4101 McEwen, Suite #800, Dallas, TX 75244 or phone them at 800-950-3415. For Allied Staffing Assistance (through MSN), please call 500-223-9230. Their website is located at www.intelistaftravel.com.

~*~

IPI Travel

IPI Travel has unlimited career opportunities in 48 states, including Hawaii and Alaska. They are JCAHO certified and offer very competitive benefits. IPI Allied is a division of Innovative Placements, offering allied health travel assignments. This division gives them the opportunity to expand their markets. They do staffing in all of the United States and Puerto Rico.

Each travel assignment is customized to fit the traveler's need: single housing, 2 bedrooms, cats, dogs, kids. They would like each of their employees to be treated like they would want to be treated. This is the golden rule we were taught while growing up. Personal service, high standards, and above-and-beyond expectations are items they strive for on a daily basis. You name it; they do it!

IPI Travel is a mid-sized company; you will always talk with your recruiter, and not an assistant. Returning phone calls is a big issue with them. They never want to hear of a recruiter not returning phone calls. Here is the deal; in order for them to be successful, their staff has to be accessible for all questions at any time. That is their motto. If a nurse goes through their system feeling like a number, they need to know about it. IPI Travel provides 24-hour emergency coverage, 7 days a week, 365 day a year. 1a.m., 2a.m., or 3 a.m., their on-call reps have the pager next to the pillow. With no more than a 30-minute lag time, your phone call will be returned.

Their company provides all the standard benefits: day-one insurance to include medical, dental, vision partner plans for medical 401-K, 3% match up to 3% of compensation (note: this is fully vested in 3 years; the 5% matching noted in the travel benefits chart are usually fully vested in 5 years), free private housing for family and pets, AAA memberships, gifts during assignments, furniture packages with flexible options, per diem options with permanent address (per government guidelines), car rentals, airfare, liability of 2 mil/4 mil (additional liability offered), free CEs license reimbursement, and $1000.00 referral bonuses. Their insurance is 2 million to 4 million in most of the country, with the exception of VA, which has increased limits; they also offer an additional insurance coverage for each traveler for a small fee.

Nurses can be on the road within two to five days, depending on the unit manager and type of nurse. If all paperwork is complete, reference checks and qualifications are in order, turn-around time could be 2 hours. This is totally situation-dependent. They could have a job for a traveler in literally hours; however, keep in mind that they will verify and check all information provided with a fine tooth comb. Quality is very important to them.

The heart and soul their staff puts into the company on a daily basis makes IPI Travel not just another “travel nurse” company. IPI Travel offers all the standard benefits, and more. The difference is that their recruiters are passionate; they live travel nursing on a daily basis, with its highs and lows. Customization—Innovative Placements believes your assignment should be not just good, but great! They hope you will have a *Wow!* factor with every aspect of your assignment.

On a daily basis, they interact with many different individuals, from the check-out lady at Wal-Mart to the CEO of a major hospital corporation. With each person the president speaks with, the one thing that remains in her mind is how each person affected them. Did the service received or given go above and beyond expectations? These are the principles Innovative Placements has maintained since 1999. To this day, they demand continued excellence from all of IPI's internal staff, as well as from their travelers. Their goal is for each of their customers to have a feeling of *Wow!* when interacting with the IPI team.

IPI achieves the *Wow!* factor with each placement by on-time delivery of completely detailed contracts, special thanks before and during the assignment, detailed housing packages, free CEs and a knowledgeable staff to help with all traveling details. In addition to all the services IPI offers, they also continue to develop client relationships throughout the United States, giving their travelers a huge network of resources and the flexibility for unlimited travel assignment choices. Each assignment is custom-designed around the traveler. IPI Travel understands healthcare professionals are in great demand; that is why they are committed to making your travel assignment rewarding and hassle-free. They guarantee that your assignment will be everything they promised. For questions regarding IP Travel or comments please feel free to call. Happy Traveling!

For more information, you can find them at 14701 Cumberland Road, Suite 350, Noblesville, IN 46060. You may also call them at 800-322-9796. Their website can be found at www.innovativeplacements.com.

~*~

Integrated Nursing Alliance

Integrated Nursing Alliance (INA) offers travel, per diem, and permanent placements in all areas of the United States for nursing and allied health professionals with the motto of "Our Nurses/ Therapists Come First." They actually limit the amount of RNs a recruiter can run on a desk so they can have free time to take care of problems and build relationships with their nurses. The average time from application to ready-to-go is about one week.

INA is medium sized. The company is going to be the difference maker in the industry. Coming from a larger company, they understand how difficult it can be working in the field and being treated like a number. Their company is going to become large, but they vow to keep the mentality of a small company that takes care of their nurses.

If the nurse has a problem at night, every one of their recruiters carries a cell phone that each nurse will have access to 24/7.

Benefits as a traveler include health insurance, paid private housing, liability insurance, travel reimbursement, continuing education reimbursement, license reimbursement, long term disability and dental insurance. Their professional liability insurance coverage is adequate, as in their company, and it covers 1 mil/3 mil aggregate. If an RN is worried that those coverages are not high enough, additional insurance can be purchased at reasonable prices.

At INA they understand that nothing is ever perfect. They know problems arise. The fact is that they are not overloaded with too many nurses on each desk because they limit the max anyone can run, which allows one to handle issues in a timely manner. Getting call-backs and resolving problems seem to be a major issue with most recruiters and companies.

Almost every recruiter at INA has come from a larger company that limited their abilities to be good recruiters. Here they all have the freedom to be flexible and help out when needed. They have all also seen what not to do because of what they have done at their previous employers.

For more information contact them at 13314 I St., Omaha, NE 68137. Phone: 888-411-4462. Website: www.inanursing.com.

~*~

Medical Express

Medical Express offers traditional travel nursing contracts that are typically 13 weeks, 36 hours per week, ,competitive pay, great housing and benefits, continuing education opportunities, allied health contracts for surg techs and respiratory therapists.

Assignments are available in all 50 states, with occasional opportunities in the United Kingdom and U.S. Virgin Islands, and they can have you ready to go in less than thirty days. The more prepared the nurse, the quicker they can get him/her started.

Although they are large, they are proud of their individualized customer service, which has been their hallmark for the 21 years they have been in business. Every traveler has a dedicated recruiter who follows that traveler from the time of application throughout his or her travel nursing experience. They have 24 hour/7 day-a-week clinical liaison support, as well as emergency on-call housing support.

Medical Express' benefits include excellent and free medical/dental insurance package, a generous 401(k) company match with immediate eligibility, free continuing education, certification reimbursement, tax-free travel reimbursement, free private housing with no hidden charges, tuition discount/reimbursement and scholarship program for nurses seeking their BSN degree, more job opportunities by far than any other company in existence, and the industry reputation of standing behind the traveler. They also provide a $2 million personal liability policy at no charge from day one of an assignment.

Their biggest pluses include their job opportunities and support, their wide variety of benefits, and most importantly, a knowledgeable, detailed, and caring personal recruiter to advise every traveler. Karena has worked for this company for over six years; the more she learns about other companies from travelers she speaks with and the longer she is involved with Medical Express the more she is convinced that she works with the best travel nursing company possible. She wouldn't go anywhere else.

For more information contact them at 1140 Westmoor Circle, Suite 325, Westminster, CO 80021 or phone them at 800-544-7255. Their website is located at www.medicalexpress.com.

~*~

Medical Solutions, Inc.

Medical Solutions offers a wide variety of travel nursing and allied health opportunities in all fifty states within the United States. They excel in personal service with their nurses and techs. The average time from acceptance of assignment to the 1st day on the job is about 2 weeks.

Referrals from travelers have led to them being one of the fastest growing staffing companies in the country. Through this rapid growth they remain committed to their main goal of treating each traveler as a person, not a number. This is the biggest difference between them and many of the other companies out there.

They are available 24 hours a day, 7 days a week. They have a pager system that will contact them with any issues after hours.

Benefits include adequate health insurance, dental insurance, paid private fully furnished housing (which includes basic cable and phone), utilities, dishes, linens and furniture.

As stated earlier, the biggest difference between Medical Solutions and the competition is their customer service. They treat each of their RNs and techs with respect, trust, honesty, and they give 100% to make sure each of their assignments is the best that it can be. Call them today! They have numerous years of experience in their recruiting and management with the travel industry. They will give you the best service and travel experiences you will ever have.

For more information, contact them at 909 North 96th Street, Omaha, NE 68114 or phone them at: 866-633-3548. The website is located at: www.MedicalSolutions.com

~*~

Medical Staffing Partners

Medical Staffing Partners Inc. (MSPI) provides travel assignments to registered nurses and surgical technicians. They are also getting more management positions for their RNs, interim clinical managers, interim house supervisors, interim DON, and case management. They have a very strong presence in the Midwest: Minnesota, North Dakota, South Dakota, Iowa, Wisconsin, and Nebraska. They also have assignments in Nevada, Wyoming, Missouri, and New York.

Ideally, the time from application to ready-to-go should be no more than a week. The factor that delays everything is how quickly the facility will interview the candidate. They work very hard to get a 24-hour commitment from the hospital; they submit the profile and they have 24 hours to speak with their candidate or choose an interview time that works for them and their candidate. Most of the clients they work for are great; however, there are always some that fall short. They communicate very closely with their professionals during this time and let them know that if they do not get called and need to move on, that is the hospital's loss.

They are a small company in which you definitely will never be treated as a number. They take pride in being a small company; they have no desire to compete with the larger corporations. They want to know their employees and learn what is important to them, professionally and personally.

Personal service is obtained by each traveler, working only with one recruiter. They all try to help their employees if they call and their recruiter is not in. They do not want to make them wait. If there is a payroll/accounting question, their professionals can speak directly with those areas.

Benefits with MSPI include 401K, medical savings account, worker's compensation, professional liability insurance, base pay of $35/hour, licensure reimbursement, airfare, rental car on many assignments, travel subsidies, and an average of $500-600 per contract. Private housing with utilities included is always provided.

What makes them different is their relationship with their employees. MSPI wants what is best for the individuals working for them. That means that if they cannot help them find what they are looking for, they will refer them to another travel company that can. They would like for travel nurses to remember that "Winters can be really fun!"

For more information contact them at 2379 Leibel Street, Suite 100, White Bear Lake, MN 55110. Their phone number is listed at 800-896-4164, and their website is listed as www.medicalstaffingpartners.com.

~*~

MedPro Staffing (formerly AbettaCare)

As of June 1st,2008, AbettaCare has officially taken the name of its parent company, MedPro Staffing. AbettaCare has been working with MedPro since 2004 and has gained recognition for being one of the top travel nursing companies.

They are very excited about this change and look forward to a seamless transition with continued success. All contact information, including the support staff and their recruiters will remain the same, only the service and the relationships that you have with your recruiter will continue to grow. In addition, MedPro staffing achieved the Gold Seal of Approval™ for health care staffing services from The Joint Commission on December 20, 2007.

At MedPro, the travelers are treated as Number 1. They pride themselves on delivering personalized service, not only through their words, but also through their actions. They spend time up front and they also do weekly follow-up calls while on assignment. This way, your recruiter gets to know each of their travelers personally, specifically asking questions about their career goals, how the assignment is going, what they have learned about the area, what challenges they have had at the hospital, what successes they have had on their assignment, etc. Your recruiter at MedPro really gains a good understanding of what's important to each particular traveler. They like to work with people through the full lifecycle of their travel healthcare career and be there for the person to service them whenever and wherever they need it. In essence, they strive for the traveler to view them as their career coach.

When MedPro approaches housing for its travelers it starts with a series of questions to find out specifically what things are important to the traveler. Things such as number of bedrooms needed, type of furniture, house-wares required, TV, washer and dryer in unit or on premises, do they have pets, anyone traveling with them, floor preference, etc. All of these questions are asked of the healthcare traveler so they can get them exactly what they need, then they communicate all of this info to the housing department and ask them to find A-Rated housing that meets the healthcare traveler's parameters. They usually provide the healthcare traveler with a couple of different options and ask him/her which one they would prefer.

MedPro provides a flexible compensation package that can be structured in any way that makes sense to the healthcare traveler. They offer either an extension or a completion bonus, whichever is more important to the healthcare traveler. For example, some travelers prefer to get the most money in their pay rate and don't care about bonuses because they are taxed so heavily. Other travelers may ask for an extra travel allowance to go home in between assignments if they are extending their contract in the same facility. The point is that they provide what's important to each individual person instead of a cookie cutter approach that does not work for everyone.

MedPro has an on call representative available 24 hours a day if a problem or emergency arises. The recruiters usually provide their travelers with their personal cell-phone in case of emergency or if they feel the urge to chat. MedPro is there to be your coach.

The reasons are many for why a nurse would prefer to travel with MedPro. That list includes weekly follow-up by a recruiter during the assignment, guaranteed personalized service defined by what the traveler tells them they need, return phone call or emailed answers to questions within a guaranteed 24 hours. They also offer a completely flexible and competitive compensation package, including a tax advantage program, free private housing, healthcare benefits (medical, dental, vision), 401K, short and long term disability, life insurance and travel reimbursement. They provide a primary point-of-contact, with a secondary back contact and no runaround to different departments and phone numbers for answers to common questions on payroll, benefits, housing, etc.

MedPro can be found at 3201 West Commercial Boulevard, Suite 116, Fort Lauderdale, Florida 33309. Phone calls can be made their toll free number: (800) 886-8108. Their website can be found at www.medprostaffing.com.

~*~

Med-Staff

Med Staff is a small company that will always treat you as an individual. In fact, they treat all of their employees as family. If you treat individuals with respect and honesty, you will find that you will have a better rapport and more long-term employees. They cover the entire United States, including Alaska and Hawaii, for travel healthcare professionals. They also provide per diem in Iowa and Illinois. Each individual is treated with respect, honesty and dignity. Each individual is unique in their own way and will be treated with individualized service.

The average time from acceptance of application to the first day on the job varies with each healthcare professional. If they are ready to travel and there is a position available, it would run no longer than 48 hours for an acceptance. If they are not ready, finishing an assignment or some other type of issue, it would have a variance.

Benefits include the insurance for the nurse to work, but if a nurse needs to obtain her own professional insurance, that is up to each individual. Yes, it is good to have this, but that is each individual's choice. Other benefits include a furnished one bedroom apartment, day one medical and dental insurance, $500.00 completion bonus, $500 travel reimbursement, Tax Advantage Plan option and an excellent payroll department.

They are dedicated to their employees and strive to make them happy and comfortable on their assignment. Their recruiters develop a rapport with each of their nurses and some have them for four years. The success of a company is the recruiter and the rapport that they develop with the healthcare professionals. They will do everything to make your travel assignment comfortable, stress free, a location where you would like to work, open communications, and an excellent payroll department. As they know, payroll can either make or break an agency. Their motto is to always be honest and upfront with each person.

Med Staff Inc. can be found at 4425 Welcome Way, Davenport, IA, 52806. You can contact them by phone at 563-359-1933 or visited on the web at www.med-staff.com.

~*~

Med Staff of Oklahoma

Med Staff of Oklahoma offers nationwide contracts with over one thousand facilities, including hospitals, clinics, corrections, out-patient and home health. Their employees can choose from several contracts, such as short-term travel, permanent placement or per diem. They are a medium-sized company, employing over 1,000 healthcare professionals nationwide, including registered nurses, licensed practical nurses, occupational and physical therapist and assistants, certified scrub techs, certified nurse aids, radiographers and lab technicians.

Personal service is a trademark of Med-Staff. As one of the few nurse-owned and operated travel companies, Med-Staff uniquely understands the field of nursing and uses this experience to better serve their employees. Med-Staff's call center is open 24/7. You will never have to leave a message on a machine when calling Med-Staff because their phone is always answered by a live person.

Med-Staff offers assignments in every state, including Hawaii and Alaska. They do not offer international assignments, however Med-Staff does offer employment for guest workers under H1-B work visas.

Med-Staff offers their fulltime employees comprehensive health insurance through one of the largest network providers in the country: Pacificare. Benefits include office co-pay, low charges for urgent care visits, prescription drug card and more. Their 401K is 100% matched up to 4% of your gross income. It also includes profit-sharing, which further increases the amount put into your account each year. They provide professional liability insurance for every travel nurse. Although there is not a need to obtain additional insurance, the nurse may obtain additional coverage for as little as $92 per year.

Typically, the turn-around for nurses who provide a complete application and the additional information, such as immunization records, skills checklist, and work history, is three-to-five business days.

MSO works for their travelers. Working conditions, assignment location, nurse-to-patient ratios and administrative support are things that other companies do not concern themselves with when placing travelers on assignments. Often times it is this attention to detail that separates the service they provide from the service of their competitors. At MSO you will never be treated like a number. They are dedicated to making your travel experience a positive one, and they pride themselves in the commitment and dedication provided to their travelers.

They can be found at 3821 East 61st, Suite 221, Tulsa, OK 74133. You may also call them at 866-787-6928 or visit them online at www.msohealth.com.

~*~

MGA Healthcare

MGA is a nationwide medical staffing company based in Phoenix, Arizona. They have been in existence since 1992. They currently have five offices throughout California, and are rapidly expanding to help fill the needs. As one of the leaders in the Medical Staffing Industries, MGA is expanding due to explosive growth in the Travel Nursing Forum. MGA offers highly competitive pay rates, housing stipends, rental car stipends, health benefits, travel reimbursements, completion bonuses and much more... They are a very unproblematic and willing company to work with and have numerous amounts of travel assignment options throughout California. They have grown their travel staff to over 150 travelers in just a few months and are seeking to continue that growth through their great reputation. They are a large enough company to fulfill all your travel needs, as well as dedicated enough to take personal care of you and any needs you may have while here in California. With offices throughout California you will always have someone to help you at any time.

Their specific regions are California and AZ. Some of their assignments are immediate and they have a nurse answer-and-assign posting and then start on Monday. Some of the responsibility relies on how fast the nurse can react to some of the paperwork, but if done promptly it can be done within 48 hours.

They are a medium-sized company, most—and they do say it with pride— of their business is from referrals. One staffer says, "I was amazed when I first started how many of my nurses were friends that recommended us." You can absolutely, without a doubt, expect personal service. The owner has taken money from his personal account to correct a pay (direct deposit) situation in order for one of his nurses to cover checks that she had written. They are most definitely available 24 hours a day!

The benefits that they provide include a friendly staff and a convenient location. They pay over what some of the larger companies are able to pay. They also offer housing stipends, rental cars, and travel arrangements.

They take their positions very seriously, while still having fun at what they do. Many of their staff have been working as account manager and/or recruiters for a while and understand the business and the problems and concerns that can arise. That is not to say that their office is all problem free, but they take on the problems in a responsible manner and take their customer service seriously, with pride, always taking into consideration and asking "what if this were me" and then dealing with the problem from that standpoint.

Most of their travelers are from referrals, which is a great sign. They have nurses that have stayed with them for the long haul, and it is a weekly occurrence that they are having some type of birthday or celebration from on of their traveling nurses. Their offices are not problem free, but they take on the problems in a responsible manner and take their customer service seriously with pride, always taking into consideration and asking "what if this were me."

For more information contact them at 990 W. 190th, Suite 410, Torrence, CA 90502, telephone them at 800-990-4642. You can check them out at www.mgahealthcare.com.

~*~

Nationwide Nurses

Nationwide Nurses (NWN) provides RNs and LPNs with ultimate personal service, unmatched in the nurse travel industry. They have assignments ranging from eight to fifty-two weeks. Nationwide Nurses has experienced travel nurses working in-house as your personal travel specialist, assuring you that you have an assignment that is custom made to fit your special wants and needs.

With a completed application, NWN can have you working in as little as three days. The average time is usually seven to ten days. This all depends on the travel distance and if the nurse has to stop along the way to get state licensure.

They offer unmatched personal service 24/7. The vice president is available anytime and answers the phones at night. They are a veteran-owned small business. You will be a name, and they will even recognize your voice.

NWN also provides housing that will accommodate you, your family and pets, if that is what you need to be comfortable during your travel assignment. They also pay all utilities, including cable TV and telephone. Other benefits include top hourly wages, guaranteed hours, weekly pay, free direct deposit, free private housing, tax free program, monthly newsletter and special gift, destination pay, upfront sign-on bonus, completion bonus, loyalty bonus, performance bonus, referral bonus, paid vacation, paid CEUs, upfront rental car, roundtrip airfare, roundtrip motel allowance, health insurance, stipend licensure paid in full, overtime available, family emergency assistance, free professional liability insurance, workers compensation, insurance incentives and other unmatched personal service. Their company carries 1 million and 6 million professional liability insurance. This is more than enough insurance for any professional. They do not believe that any nurse working for NWN will need to buy additional insurance.

They are a smaller company, by choice, so they can focus on their nurses' individual needs and concerns. They have been there for their employees for all kinds of needs. For instance, last year they had a nurse working in Arizona and his family was in Florida during the horrible hurricane season. They hired a moving van, packed their personal belongings and relocated his family to Arizona to be with him so he would not have to leave his assignment or worry about the safety of his family. Another nurse's home had been broken into while he was away working in North Mexico. They relocated his family to a safe motel and had all of the locks changed in his home. Peace of mind is priceless for their travelers, and they go above and beyond, at no cost to the nurse.

NWN staff has a tremendous retention of their travelers, and a high percentage of new employees are referred by their current travelers. That speaks volumes about them as a preferred travel nurse company.

They are located at Scenic Byway 7 South, P.O. Box 7, Marble Falls, AR 72648. They can be phoned at 866-836-8773. Their website is located at www.nationwidenurses.com.

~*~

Not Just Nurses

Not Just Nurses offers travel, per diem, and permanent placement throughout the United States. Although some of their hospitals act rapidly, there are others that are as slow as turtles. They cannot control how fast a facility responds, but they do everything possible to speed up the process. They are a small company that takes their time to get to know their nurses. They most definitely have an open-door policy!

The owner has been a nurse for about twenty-five years, so she knows what nurses like, want, and deserve. Personal service is the primary thing they do there. They hate when they are treated like a number, so they don't treat people who work with them any other way than the way they would want to be treated. Their policy is that "You get what you give in life." The owner has the office phone by her bed so, if you are desperate at 0300 and need her help—then call.

They have a laundry list of things they give their staff: health insurance, bonuses, loyalty pay, referral pay, continuing education & license reimbursement, etc. The complete list is on their website, so that anyone who is interested in all the details can take a look there.

The biggest asset with Not Just Nurses is that they are nurse owned and operated, so they really *do know* nursing. They named the company Not Just Nurses because they believe that nurses aren't "just nurses"—they are so much more! Unfortunately, they are often times highly underestimated, totally overworked and not valued as they should be by the hospitals they work for.

They suggest that they should try them on for size. They know "nurse talk," so speak! They truly have been there and done that, so they know what it's like to be in the "trenches." There aren't any "used car salesmen" hanging around there, trying to hustle the nurse. One staffer says, "The only thing I know about the hustle is—it was a disco dance!"

For more information please contact Not Just Nurses, 1624 Locust St., Norristown, PA 19401-3010, give them a call at 877-239-9700, or visit them online at www.notjustnurses.com.

~*~

Nurses PRN

Nurses PRN is a small company that specializes in temporary and contract placement of nurses in acute care and inpatient facilities such as hospitals, rehab centers, sub-acute and long-term care facilities. Nurses PRN recruits primarily for per diem and contract positions. They require all employees to have at least 1 year of current nursing experience. They are growing faster than ever and have offices in eight states. They have travel availabilities available in most parts of the U.S. All you need to do is ask! They can have you ready to go in about one week.

Personal service is what distinguishes the PRN experience. They are committed to building a personal relationship with each of their nurses and to ensure that you have all of the tools that you need to succeed! They have on-call staff available 24 hours a day, 7 days a week to assist you with any issues that arise outside of normal business hours.

They offer medical insurance to employees who average at least 30 hours per week, after 30 days of employment, as well as dental insurance, a 401k plan, holiday pay, direct deposit, referral bonus, birthday bonus, no call-in bonus, free CEUs, a uniform Store, and more.

What makes them a different company? The fact that they are at the center of their philosophy and make every attempt to inspire success by investing in their wonderful nurses. They want you to be enthusiastic about the great work that you do!

For more information you can contact them at Nurses PRN, 4321 W. College Ave., Appleton, WI 54914. Their phone number is 888-830-8811 and their website is located at www.prnhealthservices.com.

~*~

Nurses in Partnership

Nurses in Partnership (NIP) has assignments in forty-three states, education reimbursement, and possible promotion to staff, either in an operational or recruitment role. They have operational personnel that are nurses and they have a 24/7 normal and emergency service. They cover most of the USA. They also have offices in London, England; Dublin, Ireland; and Sydney, Australia. The time from interview to on-assignment varies; the fastest has been three days. Generally speaking, though, a ready-to-go nurse can expect it to take between five days and two weeks.

NIP is a medium-sized company for the travel nursing industry. They currently employ many registered nurses who have worked with them for well over two years. They receive many recommendations, especially for their understanding of clinical competencies and how they relate to the travel nurse industry.

Benefits with NIP include travel allowance, medical and dental coverage from day one, 401K (100% company match from day one for up to 4% of the nurse's salary), license reimbursement, education reimbursement, and a bonus structure that increases per assignment. Not only do they provide free private accommodations with furniture, but they are also pet friendly.

One of their greatest attributes is their industry knowledge. Executives have been in the industry for 20+ years and they understand that a travel nurse company grows only if it can retain nurses. Retention is therefore the key, and in order to retain, and therefore grow, you have to offer a "service" and you have to be accountable for that service. The nurse needs to feel that they have their best interests at heart, which only happens if they are treated as a valued member of the staff, not just another number. They care about their nurses!

For more information, you can contact them at Nurses in Partnership, 28118 Agoura Road, Agoura Hills, CA 91301 or phone them at 800-978-8555. Their website can be found at www.nipinc.com.

~*~

Nursing Innovations

Nursing Innovations (NI) is a listening, and then act-upon company. In addition to their recruiters being very accessible, they have a Nurse Advocate: Elizabeth David, RN, BSN. She was voted "nurse of the year" two years in a row at LeBonhuer Children's Hospital before she joined their staff. Elizabeth is the Florence Nightingale of NI. She is the kind of person you feel comfortable opening up to and she is available 24/7. Elizabeth is constantly sending out birthday cards and other tokens of appreciation to their nurses. A lot of their nurses also think it's cool that their AM is so accessible. She asks, "How many CEOs do you know that put their cell number on their business cards? I've worked many stressful shifts myself and completely relate to what our nurses experience."

Their insurance rates are extremely competitive and they typically pay a higher wage than many other companies. Free insurance doesn't really help if you're making significantly less per hour. I recommend that you look at the entire package, including housing, transportation, pay, and benefits.

At Nursing Innovations, you are treated like more than a number, more than a name. They currently have less than two hundred traveling nurses on assignment, with an office staff of forty. Every assignment is customized to meet your needs. Just say "no" to cookie cutter deals. They have over a thousand assignments to choose from.

They have so many options—from Magnet Facilities to Visiting Nurse Assignments—you can tell them what you are looking for and they listen, then act.

At Nursing Innovations you're the boss. They work for you! They have a great reputation among nurses and hospitals for their honesty, integrity and hard work. They have a vibrant fun and exiting corporate culture that is infectious.

For more information contact them at 6555 Quince, Suite 303, Memphis, TN 38119. You may also call them at 1-888-357-3532, or visit their website at www.NursesRock.com.

~*~

Nursing Options

Nursing Options has travel assignments nationally for RNs, LPNs, OR Techs, CCHTs and Allied Health Professionals. Most assignments are for 13 weeks, but they have the ability to customize the length of many positions. They cover all parts of the U.S., with the exception of Rhode Island.

Nursing Options is a smaller company, and they pride themselves on the personal attention they offer. They offer 24/7 support and can have you ready to go in about seven days.

Upon eligibility, Nursing Options offers flexible spending accounts, shared-cost health insurance, 401k, direct deposit, and tax advantage program. In addition, they pay the fastest referrals bonuses in the industry. Considering the minimal premium for the added professional protection, nurses should carry their own insurance. Many homeowners can endorse this coverage on their policy for less than $15/month.

Not only are they a preferred provider with many vendor management companies across the country, they also work hard to staff those areas not touched by many other travel companies.

If you're looking for options, they have many assignments unique to them.

They can be found at 215 W. Oak, 8th Floor 80521, Fort Collins, CO 80525. To learn more, visit www.NursingOptions.com or call 877-Nurse-50.

~*~

Nursing Ventures

Nursing Ventures is a small-to-medium sized company that has extremely high paying opportunities for Nursing and Allied Healthcare Professionals. They offer local per diem, local contracts, travel assignments and permanent placement. Although they do not offer any international services, they do cover all of the United States, including Alaska and Hawaii. They can get you going in one or two weeks, depending on the responsiveness of the applicant. Their personal service includes after-hours support for their employees and hospital clients. Their toll free number will direct after-hours callers to their administrator on call.

The number one benefit from working with Nursing Ventures is the exceptionally high pay. They are against any type of program, vendor, or overhead that will decrease the bottom line of their employees. They do not offer referral bonuses, "free private housing," transportation, completion bonuses, free laptops, free scrubs, stethoscopes, health insurance or anything else that will take money out of the checks their nurses work so hard for. Nursing Ventures believes that hard working professionals can manage their money better than they can.

Nursing Ventures Inc. is a dedicated professional temporary healthcare staffing company whose primary goal is to pay their employees as much as possible. In their 4 year history they have never *found any* other staffing company that can beat their high pay rates, based on the same billing rate. They are creating a huge niche between the large greedy publicly traded staffing companies and the small "mom and pop" or internet "start your own nurse agency for $299" companies. The owners of Nursing Ventures Inc. are all RN's who work full time for client facilities alongside their employees. They do not rely on their employees for their bread and butter. The owners of Nursing Ventures Inc. believe that the time for change in the temporary healthcare staffing industry starts with them, and it starts now. Nurses have been taken advantage of for years by large staffing companies that are making huge profits from the hard work of nurses like us. Nursing Ventures Inc. will change that! They are against corporate greed and against small get-rich-quick companies that know nothing about the staffing industry or employment law. Nursing Ventures Inc. has elected to take the high road—the path of professionalism and integrity for all healthcare professionals who choose to have more freedom in their careers. Their employees understand that their careers are tools that allow them to live life the way they want to, on their terms and not working five to seven days a week just to make ends meet. Nursing Ventures Inc. is outraged by the huge profit margins that are taken from the billing rates charged to the hospital clients in return for the hard work of nursing professionals who should be getting paid double what they are making.

Nursing Ventures Inc. is a professional healthcare staffing company whose goal is to pay their employees more than any other staffing company, period! They are not a staffing company that is right for everyone. They seek healthcare professionals who want to make the most of their time so they can live their lives as they choose. Nurses are human beings, not wage/insurance slaves who are locked into a cycle of work/pay bills-work/pay bills. Nursing Ventures Inc. is about blocking anything that reduces the hourly pay for their employees' bottom line. Work to live, *not* live to work.

Nursing Ventures can be found at 2825 East Cottonwood Parkway, Suite 500, Salt Lake City, UT 84121. Their phone number is 877-657-6262. Or you can visit them online at www.nursingventures.com.

~*~

PPR Healthcare

PPR offers travel opportunities for RNs and Allied Health across the US. They also have an International Department for bringing nurses into the US. Their recruiters are very knowledgeable and can help you with any assignment in the United States, including Alaska or Hawaii. They can have nurses interviewed, offered, and ready to go in as little as a week, depending on the quickness of the facility and the nurse to complete the paperwork.

They are a medium-sized company and strive to put their nurses first by offering first-class service. The nurse is never just a number. The recruiter-to-nurse ratio is very low. Each recruiter works with a small amount of nurses. Recruiters offer the use of their personal cell phones for emergencies after hours.

Benefits include health, dental, life, vision, short-term and long-term disability, 401K, loyalty bonuses, free private fully furnished housing and 100% utilities, 100%licensure reimbursement, and a whole lot more.

Their service is top-notch; they believe that this is what separates them from the others. They offer flexible benefits, meaning that they gear their package according to what is most important for each nurse.

For more information, PPR can be found at 333 First Street North, Suite 200, Jacksonville Beach, FL 32250, or phone them at 888-909-5038. Their website can be found at www.pprhealthcare.com.

~*~

Premier Healthcare Professionals

Premier Healthcare Professionals Inc. (PHP) is part of a large group of companies, specializing in the placement of nurses and other healthcare professionals around the world. The group has company-owned offices in London, Sydney and Johannesburg, and it is from these offices that it places nurses throughout the UK, Australia and South Africa.

They arrange professional liability insurance for each of their nurses at no cost to the individual. The insurance is for the sole benefit of their nurses, and they have coverage for each nurse at any of their client facilities. The cover is automatically included within the comprehensive benefits package that they provide to their nurses.

All of their nurses are provided with a toll free number that can be used to contact a PHP representative 24 hours of the day. PHP prides itself on the level of service they provide their nurses and is more than happy to deal with any issues that may arise, day or night.

The PHP group has been placing nurses in the US for nearly two decades. They understand the professional and personal requirements of each of their nurses, and furthermore, they fully respect each and every one of those requirements. Most members of their recruitment and placement staff have worked with the PHP Group for more than 8 years and are fully aware of the importance of their nurses' personal satisfaction. They are very proud of the fact that over 85% of their new enquiries originate from referrals from past or present working nurses. The business simply would not have grown to the force it is today, through the many market changes, without its dedicated and experienced team of staff members.

In addition to providing unparalleled service standards to their nurses, they also boast the most flexible benefits package available in the market today. They allow all of their nurses to choose from a menu of benefits and pay rates to match their own personal requirements. They guarantee to at least match any legitimate pay and benefits package available in the marketplace today. Their nurses appreciate the personal service and pay and benefits that they offer to them and this is evidenced by the fact that some of their nurses have been contracted with their group companies for almost a decade.

For more information contact Premier Healthcare Professionals, 2450 Atlanta Hwy, Suite 601 Cumming, GA 30040, Phone: (866) 296 3247, Fax: (866) 666 2622, or visit their website at www.travelphp.com.

~*~

PRN Health Service

PRN Health Service provides staffing opportunities for all medical specialties, including LPN, RN, and Techs for travel, per diem, or permanent placement in all fifty states. They consider all who work with them as their friends. They try to treat every worker as they would want to be treated. Their major benefit is that they are a company that is built on integrity.

While all nurses that are employed by them are covered, as a friend, they personally encourage all to carry personal policies. The cost is reasonable, and they feel it is added protection, peace of mind, plus it opens up more opportunities for nurses.

They are very small, which is why they originally chose PRN to work with. They feel personally responsible for every nurse who works with them; they see to it that they have a good assignment and are well taken care of.

Their main office number has a recorder on after hours, which rolls to a pager, so if someone leaves a message it is answered immediately. Their offices are in their homes, so they are available most of the time, including weekends and holidays. They will get the nurse there the next day if needed. It just depends on the start date, where they are located, and what is more convenient for the nurse.

The owners of PRN are both travel nurses. They are soldiers in the field also. More importantly, they are small enough that they have the flexibility to work with each nurse individually as to what they need. They do not work off of commission, which is normally how many companies pay their recruiters; therefore, they have no financial gain for placing nurses. They actually enjoy what they do! Working to get a nurse an assignment where he or she wants, with the best possible rate they can give, is the reward.

The recruiters live in small rural towns, and work with a small company by choice. They are friends, while at work or home. They consider nurses who work with them as their friends also. They are not a large corporation, nor are they owned by one. They try to build friendships, not careers. The most valuable resource a company has is the people who work for it. If you treat each person individually, with respect and accountability, your company builds itself.

For more information you can snail mail them at PRN Health Service, P.O. Box 10546, Enid, OK 37306 or phone them at 866-830-0003. Their website can be found at www.prntravelnurse.com.

~*~

Professional Care Health Services

Professional Care Health Services are presently contracting correctional nursing in California, with some Home Health in Chicago, Illinois. Their company is a very small company that treats their nurses as individuals, yet they try to offer as much as the big leaguers with their competitive rates. Presently they are licensed to do business in Illinois, California, Georgia and Oregon.

The Chief Executive Officer is an RN and a previous traveler. She personally gives others what she would want, if at all possible. Because she is owner and CEO of this business she makes the final decisions without all the red tape. Being a night owl, she is often the one who answers the phone at night.

They start to work on the application after she talks to the nurse who is interested in the assignment and is confirmed and they receive his/her credentials. When they have an open assignment they do not delay in trying to fill the position.

They can offer individual plan health insurance in which they negotiate a sharing of the cost. The plan is designed so you can take it with you if you want to move on. Also, life insurance is available, as well as 401k for long-term employees. They do have a vacation gift for those who have been employed with them for one consistent year. The CEO makes sure that the professional malpractice coverage they carry is good enough for the nurses she employs. For that reason, she maintains a nurse as an employee and deducts taxes. However, there is nothing wrong with carrying your own personal coverage; the cost is pennies on the dollar.

The personal relationship that the CEO establishes with each nurse is the reason PRCS is different. She cares about the traveler's concerns to make the assignment a good match.

Feel free to call them with any questions about the company. The website is a great place to get basic information, but it isn't always kept up-to-date. They look forward to placing some of their nurses in the near future. They presently have some openings in CA Corrections.

For more information they can be found at 3007 Panola Road, Suite C-214, Lithonia, GA 30038, or contact can be made through telephone at 866-418-9393. Their website can be found at www.professionalcarehealthsvcs.com.

~*~

Professional Respiratory Care Services

PRCS offers travel assignments to Registered Nurses and Respiratory Therapists nationwide, with their focus on the great southwest: Phoenix, Las Vegas, San Diego, and Hawaii. They do not offer international assignments, but they do employ international nurses. Depending on the traveler's availability and timeframe, PRCS can process a nurse's application and get the nurse working in about a week.

Personal service is an absolute with them! PRCS is locally owned and managed by a healthcare clinician. Their travel manager is also a healthcare clinician. Their corporate office is located in Phoenix. They also have a satellite office in Las Vegas. Their telephones are answered 24 hours a day, 365 days per year. Their travelers and hospital clients can reach them at any time. Even their managers are available to address issues around the clock.

PRCS is a small organization. Their owner and travel manager are both healthcare clinicians. They pride themselves in getting to know their nurses and therapists on an individual basis. They treat all of their nurses as individuals with specific personalities, needs, and attention.

PRCS offers top pay, guaranteed hours, uncapped travel reimbursement, licensure reimbursement, free private furnished housing, completion bonuses, and benefit package as of the first day of assignment. The professional liability insurance they provide is sufficient to cover their traveling professionals. A great benefit to Canadian-educated nurses is that PRCS will reimburse the cost of your NCLEX exam.

PRCS is unique in that they are owned and managed by healthcare clinicians and that they are local. Their travelers will personally know them and receive the personal attention they deserve. They value and appreciate their nurses and look forward to continued working with them!

For more information you can write to them at Professional Respiratory Care Services Inc., 3801 N. 24th Street, Phoenix, AZ 85016 or phone them at 602-508-1000. Their website is located at www.prcshealthcare.com.

~*~

Pro-Med Staffing

Pro-Med Staffing is dedicated to serving your best interest whether that may be career aspirations, location choice, or making sure that your achievements are recognized and rewarded appropriately. Therefore, they will work with you every day in every way to insure that your goals and dreams are met.

Since they realize that everyone is different they try to be attentive to those differences when targeting the right position for you. They try to get to know each and every one personally so they can customize their benefit program to meet your needs.

When dealing with Pro-Med you can have confidence in knowing that you are working with people of integrity who care and are sensitive and competent to work for you. An added benefit is that they are small enough to give you lots of individual attention, which includes being able to talk directly with the owner or the Human Resources Director. They can and have turned applications around in less than 24 hours, but the typical time is 24-72 hours.

Benefits include top hourly pay and excellent overtime/holiday compensation, free first day of health insurance coverage with a national carrier plus coverage for dependent(s) with deductions for additional individual(s), generous housing allowance, direct deposit of pay weekly, $500 completion bonus from Pro-Med Staffing at the completion of each thirteen (13)-week assignment, pass through of hospital bonus (if offered), 401K availability with Pro-Med Staffing contribution, referral fee when anyone you refer completes his/her first assignment with Pro-Med, customized benefits, customer service 24/7, and individual attention beyond compare.

Their home office is in Phoenix, Arizona and they have successfully placed R.N.'s in fifteen different states. Pro-Med has been a member of the Arizona Hospital and Healthcare Association (AzHHA) for over eight years.

For more information you can contact them at Pro-Med Staffing, Inc., P.O. Box 51855, Phoenix, AZ 85076, local Phoenix # 480-496-7111, toll-free # 800-980-9070, website www.pro-medstaffing.com.

~*~

Qshift Travel Nurses

Qshift offers travel healthcare placement for nurses, technologists and therapists throughout the United States. Their assignments are typically 13 weeks long, but they can be as short as eight weeks or as long as the facility and traveler would like to extend them. If the facility would like to hire the traveler regular full time, they are able to favorably respond to that request as well. Their goal is to meet the needs of the facilities, as well as those of their travelers. Their employees reach them live 24/7/365 days a year. If the need is to talk to their recruiter or placement coordinator, they will connect them. There are no recordings or message banks at qShift Travel Nurses.

Personal service is the only kind of service they offer. Qshifts's foundation is based on advocacy. Their company's foundation is sterling service and advocacy. Personal service and commitment to their employees and client facilities is their standard mode of business.

They serve approximately 40 states and have 800 to 1000 open requests at any given time. They are not as large as the largest agencies; however, they have as many requests. They look forward to continued exponential growth due to their philosophy. QShift applications may be completed by mail, or Internet based. The process is very quick and dependent on the timely receipt of a completed profile to begin the process. Once they have a profile to go through their processes they are in contact with the individual almost daily to complete the final documents. They are very aggressive in promoting and facilitating the interview. Once the facility and employee agree to terms, a start date is verified. As a rule, from interview to first day on the job will be anywhere between three days to two weeks. This time can be shortened, but they will work very closely with the traveler to ensure that they have a quick turnaround on all documents required to begin an assignment.

They are a small-to-medium sized company in which no employee is treated as a number. You will always be treated by name; they don't issue numbers for their travelers. They continually have new employees who express that is how they had felt. Service is not rocket science; it is merely one commitment at a time to one person at a time. This is QShift Travel Nurses.

Travelers are beginning to realize that all significant travel companies have the same benefits; the difference is in how they are presented. It is important that travelers listen closely to what is actually being said. If there is a primary difference in qShift employees it is in the allocation of non-taxable compensation. At like locations and positions, QShift employees will receive more net pay after taxes than most other companies provide. Their interest is in maximizing the take-home pay of their employees. They always follow the federal guidelines to the maximum allowance for the employees' benefit. Their employees appreciate the difference. Other benefits include weekly direct deposit, 401k with matching funds, bonuses (application, assignment, loyalty, referral), license reimbursement, continuing education reimbursement, free medical, free life insurance with medical insurance, dental and vision insurance (section 125), travel reimbursement, and tax-free weekly stipend. For housing, they offer private one-bedroom, corporate housing or a housing stipend, whichever will work best for the traveler. Professional liability insurance is the traveler's decision. They do have general and professional liability insurance that covers the traveler while on assignment for Qshift that they feel is sufficient. They do not encourage nurses to have double coverage if they have never had a litigious situation. Their insurances are comprehensive and exhaustive, so nurses do not need to get their own. They recommend that they not waste their money if they inquire about it. Double insurance is for insurance companies' and attorneys' benefit. For over 16 years Qshift has never had litigation directly against any employees due to quality assurance or quality and professionalism. If the need arises, their nurses know to let them address and solve any issue.

Their employees make them a better company. They are the purveyor of their service and brand. Qshift Travel Nurses foundation is "service and advocacy." Qshift is not in this business solely for the profits they derive. They incorporate the highest standards of business integrity and honorable ethics, the focus of their administrative/office staff to their field employees. This in turn lends itself to a healthy hospital through a satisfied community. The profits received are as they should be—"divided equally." When you see a Qshift employee, watch and learn from them as they do their job! Their foundation, their service oriented culture, their recruiters, their business practices, their systems and the way they advocate for their travelers also makes a big difference. Even though their travelers may be all over the country, they strive to make them feel right at home with them in Colorado.

They look forward to visiting with everyone interested in complete support and advocacy with the highest compensation packages available across the nation in apples-to-apples comparisons. They are here for you, and you will know you are receiving exactly what you expected. It starts with their commitment to each person. They realize that their success is the result of the travelers they have and the hospitals they serve. They never take either for granted and realize that they have to "earn" their business. They work hard every day, every interaction, to make sure they satisfy their travelers and their client hospitals.

They do this by having honest, clear communications and by fulfilling their promises. Call them today; you won't be disappointed.

Their offices are located at 214 E. Monument Street, Colorado Springs, CO 80919. You can contact them by phone at 800-733-6877, or visit their website at www.qshift.com.

~*~

Quik Travel Staffing

Quik Travel Staffing specializes in dialysis travel staffing and services all major dialysis healthcare providers. They are a medium-sized company with a small business attitude where every contract counts. They cover the entire continental US, as well as Hawaii. They can have a nurse on the road within two days. Personal service is a "yes, yes, yes, yes" with their company, and they are available 24/7.

Benefits include a 401K plan, a referral bonus, completion bonus, express pay, direct deposit, free travel, housing, local transportation and much more, including plenty of professional liability insurance.

They are privately owned and highly specialized in dialysis. They believe that their nurses, as well as their clients, are their customers, and that they have to bend over backwards to stay competitive in this marketplace. This practice made them the leader in the dialysis staffing industry.

For more information call them today at 800-544-2230. They can be found at 150 E. Olive Ave, Suite 308, Burbank, CA 91502 or found online at www.qtstaffing.com.

~*~

The Right Solutions

The Right Solutions offers a wide range of opportunities all across the US. They have assignments that vary from 4-26 weeks. They have Corp, State, VA, and Indian Hospitals. They treat every nurse like a personal friend, because that is what they are.

They have assignments in just about every state. They have a contract with the government to staff all of the VA Hospitals, military bases, and Indian hospitals as well. This leaves the possibilities endless. They are currently working on getting contracts internationally. From the time of assignment selection until the time the nurse is set to go sometimes is very quick. They have a lot of "quick starts." They submit and get a start date of the next week, or sometimes even the same week.

They are a medium sized company with all of their nurses treated as personal friends. Most of the recruiters send gifts and/ or cards for a number of reasons, whether it is the start of a new assignment, a birthday, or an illness. Their owner is very involved with their nurses. She has an "open door" policy and anyone can speak to her at any time.

They have an on-call manager who can be reached 24 hours a day. Most of the recruiters also give out their personal numbers so they can call them if they need to talk too. If you are lonely or your car breaks down, you know you can call them.

They give a travel allowance to and from assignments. They have a referral program that offers bonuses. They do license reimbursement. They have personal insurance. They also have an IRA that you can invest in from day one. The list goes on and on. Their professional insurance is great, and usually nurses do not need to obtain their own.

They are owned by a nurse, and she is someone that is there for you. You are not just a number, but a person—a personal friend. They care about their "family" that is out there in a strange new place. Not only do they want to know your thoughts, but they listen and take what you have to say to heart. They would love to talk with all of you and get to know you and your needs.

The Right Solution can be contracted at 311 Henri De Tonti Blvd, Tontitown, AR 72770 or called at 888-987-8233. Their website is located at www.therightsolutions.com.

~*~

Rn Demand

Rn Demand has nationwide eight-to-thirteen-week travel nursing opportunities. Over 20 years of staffing, every specialty in a hospital does not just happen without customer service or lots of hard work. They cover the entire U.S and have a regionalized marketing focus; this means more people creating more opportunities. They are not international. They can have new providers ready in about two weeks, unless they put a rush on it, and for a provider who has worked for them before it is about one day.

They started with the nursing division in its infancy and have watched it grow. Comparatively, they are probably still small, and their 3-pronged approach allows them to pay more attention to detail. They know every nurse's name that works for them. They also have a 24-hr. 30-minute call-back pledge. Their working providers have an emergency pager number where someone can always be reached.

In addition to their free insurance, free fully-furnished housing, day-one insurance, $1000 referral bonus, and weekly direct deposit, they pay for and process your licenses on the front end and will get you future licenses. They have a 1 million/6 million dollar policy that should be sufficient for an RN. The only specialty they might recommend supplement coverage for would be in the O.R. or O.B fields.

They have a three-pronged approach to business. They have regionalized marketers who focus on bringing in jobs, an account representative that handles all of the logistics while on assignment, and a recruiter who only has your interest in mind. They are separated like this because it makes each of them experts at what they do. RN Demand is still in the process of growing, but one day they want to be the company every hospital turns to and every nurse wants to work for.

Their company can be found at 5001 Statesman Drive, Irving, TX 75063 or they can be telephoned at 866-616-0266. Their website is located at www.rndemand.com.

~*~

RN & RT Temps

RN and RT Temps provide interim staffing and permanent placement for all nursing and allied health professionals. You will always have a live person to speak with and will not be stuck with a voice prompter or messaging system.

They cover the entire United States, the U.S. Virgin Islands, and some international assignments through the federal government. Assuming that the nurse complies with JCHAO guidelines in terms of supplying them with the proper documentation for the employee file, they would be able to place the nurse in 24 hours. They are a medium-sized company where their recruiters will always remember you by name, and they have a recruiter on call 24 hours per day.

RN & RT Temps also offer medical, dental, vision, prescription, long-term and short-term disability, paid housing and travel, 401k, and much more. The nurse will be fully covered through their malpractice, workman's comp, and general liability coverage.

The company was founded by a healthcare professional in 1987 who happens to be very involved with the day-to-day operations and has a wealth of industry knowledge. "Staffing with you in mind" is their motto and mission.

For more information, they can be found at 9 West Front Street, Media, PA 19063, or you may call them at 800-677-8233. Their websites can be found at www.rttemps.com and www.rntemps.com.

~*~

Rn Recruit

Rn Recruit offers four to thirteen week travel contracts to healthcare professionals. They cover the United States, even though at this time they do not have assignments in all states, they will go after a specific hospital if the traveler requests, to try to place the traveler where they want to work next. They can have you ready to go in about four days.

They are a medium company who lives by the golden rule of doing unto others what they would like to have done to them. They strive to be the best and not the largest travel company. Part of that is why they provide a twenty-four hour clinical person on call for clinical situations and any emergency that arises.

Some of the benefits of working for Rn Recruit include weekly pay, direct deposit, tax-advantage, 401K, medical insurance and short-term assignments.

They are different from other travel companies due to their first-hand experience of nurse traveling. They work full time at ensuring that they remain the exception to the rule for travelers.

For more information you can contact them at 774 May's Blvd #10, Suite 481, Incline Village, NV 89451 or phone them at 866-466-2721. Their website is located at www.rnrecruit.com.

~*~

RN Travel Connection

RN Travel Connections offers eight to thirteen week travel assignments for RNs and Allied Health across the United States. A $1000 vacation bonus is available after completion of three consecutive thirteen-week assignments; a $500 minimum completion bonus is available per 13-week assignment. They have positions across the entire United States for RNs with at least 2 years of experience; they belong to every state association that is contracting.

Personal service is a must! They email mapquest directions for their nurses, showing the destination they are going to, where they are staying, and to the hospital. Your recruiter will contact you weekly to see how things are going. All assignments offer a minimum $500 completion bonus; $1000 bonus is paid after completion of three assignments, 401K with $1/$1 match up to 6% of pay and United Healthcare PPO with drug card and dental starting on day one. An RN is on call 24 hours a day.

They are a medium, and yes, they will know you as a name, from recruiting to payroll to housing to quality assurance to the staffing and marketing departments, who will be submitting your information to the hospitals when you are ready to interview. All forms needed are on line at their website. Payroll is weekly; if they don't get your timeslip, they will call you. If you look on Delphi you won't find anything bad about their company. They treat their nurses great. If you want to talk to one of their current travelers for a reference they can set that up.

Many different bonuses, including referral, completion, extra hours completion, $1000 vacation bonus after 3 assignments, a great 401K plan with $1/$1 match up to 6% through the Hartford group, your own furnished apartment with electric paid up to $100/month, all deposit fees—unless you have a pet and they prorate that over the 13-week contract, weekly pay, direct deposit, tax-free per diem program for nurses who qualify, personalized attention, paid drug screen and titers, and licensure reimbursement. The company professional insurance they have takes care of everything. If the nurse has her own professional insurance, any actions will be filed against the nurse's insurance and theirs, but if the nurse doesn't have insurance the company is 100% liable.

They can tell you the rates for different states up front, along with all of their benefits, but they need the application and skills checklist before they can submit you to the hospital. Average time can be from 1 week, if you can get your information in, up to 3 weeks. All forms are online.

They are nurse-owned and operated, along with a commitment to "make things right" for their nurses. Most of their nurses continue to work for them because they can find them the locations they like and where they know they will take care of them.

What would they like travelers to know? Never start an assignment with a company without a signed contract. Their standard contract is online if you want to review it. RN Travel Connection will take care of you. Celebrate and promote Nursing!

You can contract Rn Travel Connection at 8255 E. Raintree, Suite 100, Scottsdale, AZ 84260 or phone them at 800-243-5939. Their website can be found at www.rntravelconnection.com.

~*~

RTG Medical

RTG Medical offers both travel and permanent placement opportunities in nearly all areas of the medical field all across the United States, but they have not ventured into international assignments at this point.

RTG offers unmatched customer service and they focus on developing personal relationships with all of their employees. Their motto is "People Are Our Only Asset." Employees work with only one recruiter who handles all of the details involved with employment, paying special attention to each employee's personal needs. The average time from application to assignment can be as little as five to seven days. This is really up to the nurse and how quickly they can get to the assignment.

They are a smaller company with about thirty recruiters, growing at a rapid pace. They are focused on never growing too quickly and will always make sure that their employees are never just a number. An RTG Medical Recruiter is available 24 hours a day, 7 days a week.

Benefits include health, dental, and life insurance, 401K, referral bonuses, loyalty bonuses, rental car, and roundtrip airfare. Their professional liability insurance is adequate enough to work under without any concern.

RTG Medical separates itself with the personal service that they offer to their employees on a daily basis. They also make sure that they always follow through on what they say they are going to do. They are JCAHO Certified and recently named by *Inc. Magazine* as one of the "Top 500 Fastest Growing Privately Held Companies" in the United States.

For more information they can be found at 1005 E. 23rd Street, Suite 200, Omaha, NE 68025, or can be reached by phone at 866-784-2329. They can be found online at www.rtgmedical.com.

~*~

Sagent Healthstaff

Sagent Healthstaff offers travel and local contracts to all nurse specialists and allied health professionals. Regional markets offer daily per diem positions for both professional groups. Their company builds and develops regional markets to improve service and support to their healthcare professionals and client facilities. Sagent Healthstaff's current regional offices include Northeast, Mid-Atlantic, Southeast, and Pacific. Sagent does offer travel contracts outside these regions also. They can have you ready to go in a week or less. Most client hospitals start new contracts on Mondays.

Sagent Healthstaff is a small-to-medium sized company. No matter what size they are, everyone is a name. Sagent prides themselves on the personal services they provide to all their candidates, employees, and even past employees, at every level. Personal healthcare is an absolute. They know that service and support (to employees and clients) are greatly improved by offering stronger regional support, rather than a single national approach. They invest in opening regional offices to insure that their services are met with the greatest satisfaction. This approach has resulted in their growth by over 100% each year, and in 2005 they grew over 200%. They have 24/7 on-call services and a Sagent staff member is always available.

Their benefits include day-one no cost medical and dental insurance, 401k participation tax advantage program, travel reimbursement up to $500, 100% license reimbursement, free private housing or housing subsidy, credentialing assistance, CEU program, weekly pay, direct deposit, reimbursement for Visa screen and NCLEX-RN exam, professional liability insurance, and 24/7 customer support. Their professional insurance covers 100% of all active Sagent Healthstaff employees.

Sagent Healthstaff differs by their regional geographic approach. Most other travel firms offer a single national approach. Sagent results include (1) Regional recruiting teams that identify assignments that best suit traveler needs; (2) Offer greater understanding of the facility and region where their travel employees work and live; (3) Regional support, as opposed to a single national approach. The Sagent Healthstaff team possesses over 75 years of industry knowledge. They are a dedicated group that works to keep ahead of the travel industry and they lead with a philosophy to "give travelers more," and they design their business to exceed travelers' financial goals and meet their personal needs.

For more information contact them at 460 Totten Pond Road, Suite 370, Waltham, MA 02454 or phone them at 877-447-3376. Their website can be found at www.sagenths.com.

~*~

Sedona Medical Staffing

Sedona Medical Staffing supplies hospitals nationwide with qualified RN's, LPN's and all areas of Allied Health. When working with Sedona Medical Staffing you will be guaranteed one-on-one service. Their recruiters have developed an excellent rapport with their healthcare employees, and every Friday they will contact them to make sure that their assignment is going ok, see if there is anything they need, and to just say hello.

They have assignments all over the United States, including Alaska and Hawaii, and can have you going within one or two weeks on the average. This will vary, as we all know, with each hospital and their different protocols to their acceptance of an application and the placement of a position.

They are a medium-sized company, and their recruiters will treat you as an individual, with respect and honesty, and they will contact you every Friday to see how everything is going with you. They will become your friend and not just your employer. They also have a twenty-four/seven customer service to assist their employees. We all know that issues do not come between the hours of 8am and 4pm, so they have instilled this strict policy.

They provide day one health and dental insurance, private furnished one bedroom apartment, $500.00 completion bonus, a $500.00 referral bonus, and a $500.00 travel reimbursement. They have weekly pay through direct deposit through their outstanding payroll department.

Sedona Medical feels that each individual is unique, has different needs and should be treated with respect and honesty. They strive to make each health professional feel that they are being assisted on a one-to-one basis. Their benefits are excellent and they follow through with what they indicate that they will do for each individual. They believe the following: "See the United States with an agency that cares for you. Stop working for the agencies and let the agency work for you."

You can find them at 610 Valley View Drive in Moline, IL 61265, or phone them at 800-730-9060. Their websiite is located at www.sedonamedical.com.

~*~

Select Medical Staffing

Select Medical Staffing offers short-term, long-term, travel, and per diem assignments. They recognize the importance of recruiting/retaining outstanding healthcare professionals. They appreciate having the opportunity to work for you. They currently have assignments in Louisiana, Texas, and Mississippi and can have you ready to go in one week.

They are a medium-sized nursing agency. Each and every employee is important to them. They pride themselves on developing long professional relationships. Nurses can reach their recruiter or clinical supervisor 24/7.

Benefits include premium pay rates, daily pay, direct deposit, great housing or a healthy housing stipend, dental and health benefits, 401K, travel pay with bonuses and outstanding customer service 24 hours a day, 7 days a week, and 365 days a year. They provide adequate professional liability insurance for their nurses; however, they recommend that nurses obtain additional coverage.

They are dedicated healthcare professionals that know and appreciate that you have many choices when it comes to choosing a travel company. They work hard to find the right assignment for you.

Founded by Critical Care RN's, their management has been representing professionals like you for over 10 years. They are looking for outstanding healthcare professionals who are ready, willing and able to enjoy high salaries, interesting assignments and professional independence.

For more information you can contact them at 19376 N. 9th Street, Suite 100, Covington, LA 70433. Their phone number is 800-783-9294, and their website can be found at www.selectmedicalstaffing.com.

~*~

Soliant Health

Soliant Health provides thirteen-week assignments in nursing, respiratory therapy, and physical therapy for locations throughout the United States. They are a medium-sized company through which you can expect excellent personal service.

Benefits that they provide include weekly payroll, Blue Cross/ Blue Shield insurance, dental insurance, vision insurance, and personal service. Even at night they have an answering service that contacts managers if there is a problem after hours.

Their personal service and turnaround of about ten days from application to on the job makes them more than just another company.

To find out more you can give them a call at 800-866-0852 or visit them at 1979 Lakeside Parkway, Suite 250, Tucker, GA 30084 or visit their website at www.soliant.com

~*~

StaffingMedical USA

StaffingMedical USA (SMUSA) has travel nursing positions for RNs across the entire USA. They can have you ready to go in seven to twenty-one days and you always get service with a smile! Risk management is also available 24/7 if needed.

You are treated as a name at SMUSA; they are like family to their nurses. That said, they are a smaller company, but they have gained much exposure lately with their excellent opportunities.

They provide both liability and major medical insurance free to the nurse. Dental and vision insurance along with 401k, Aflac, workman's comp. insurance. Their professional liability insurance policy is one of the best out there, but a nurse having her own insurance as well is a good idea.

That personal touch and willingness to please that all nurses look and strive for in a company makes them stand out in a crowd. Have fun on the road and work hard, but most of all enjoy!

For more information they can be found at 15849 N. 71st Street #100, Scottsdale, AZ 85252 or be phoned at 877-280-2600. They are online at www.staffingmedical.com.

~*~

TaleMed

TaleMed offers a wealth of traveling nurse employment opportunities all across the country. From friendly towns to exciting facilities to bustling metropolitan centers, they can place you in the locations and nursing jobs that you have always dreamed of, and from the community facility to the prestigious teaching hospital they can find the professional environment that's just right for you. TaleMed reaches into all fifty states, offering a wealth of traveling nurse job opportunities, and they can have you ready to go between 24 hours and 4 days for a nurse that is ready to work and has completed all the necessary details prior to submitting to a hospital.

They are a small company. You are absolutely 100% treated as a name, and they will be on a first-name basis with you. Personal and exceptional service is what they strive for. As a nurse and as their employee, you are their number one priority. You have access to their personal cell phone numbers. They also have a "hotline" of somebody on call each night. It is critical to them that you know that they are available at all times for you.

They offer paid benefits that start from day one. This includes medical, dental, AD&D, life and prescription coverage. They also have made available short and long term disability. 401K is also available. 100% of your malpractice is covered by TaleMed.

At TaleMed they understand that traveling to the leading hospitals and exciting locations is a big attraction to the job. The new challenges and new opportunities to grow in your profession are just as important. Or perhaps you want to focus on your work and your life, leaving the hassles and headaches behind. They have listened, and they've built a company that works hard for you and your dreams.

At TaleMed you don't work for them; they work for you. TaleMed is built on experience and knowledge in the medical field. With over 75 years of experience supporting their goal and service, they make you their number one priority.

For more information you can contact them at 403 Loveland Madeira Road, Loveland, Oh 45140, or talk to them at 800-494-0087. They can be found online at www.talemed.com.

~*~

Tech Group

Tech Group staffs radiation therapy, radiology, sonography, nursing and laboratory. They offer travel, per diem, temp to perm and perm opportunities throughout the United States.

If you are "ready-to-go"—as in your paperwork is in order, you are licensed and packed—they can get you on the road in a matter of days. A week is more typical; although, they have a lot of flying out on Friday to start on Monday. It depends on how adventurous you are.

Tech Groups is a small company that has been in business for over seventeen years. They are based in Spokane, WA. They were started by health care professionals who also have traveled. Not only do they know your name, they know your dog's name and how they are doing in obedience school. They know only know your child's name, but how they are doing in school and whether or not they will be traveling with you. They take pride in knowing their travelers and their needs. That is the only way they can make the great match and make a great assignment to remember.

It is their mission to provide the highest quality patient care. They do that by finding and retaining the highest quality health care providers. They are about people and they strive to exceed your expectations. A big part of that is to offer personal service to their travelers. They know what it's like to be on the road, away from home and family. They are happy to make special arrangements for housing: top floor for a day sleeper or bottom floor for a mom who uses a walker, finding pet-friendly housing or remembering birthdays, anniversaries, holidays and special occasions.

They have a staffing coordinator on call twenty-four hours a day, seven days a week. They are a small company and they share working space. They all know each other's travelers and take time at the end of each day to review who is traveling or moving or picking up a car or...well, you get the idea.

Tech Groups offers top pay, shift differentials and weekend differentials, per-diem, free, private housing, auto allowances or rentals, covered travel. They also offer referral bonuses, hours of service bonuses, continuing education reimbursement. They offer

401K, medical and dental insurance, long and short term disability and life insurance—and more.

They are a small company with a big heart. They strive to exceed your expectations. Many of their travelers have traveled with them for many assignments because they can feel the difference. They appreciate their travelers and want to make sure that they know it. Tech Group loves to think out of the box to make great healthcare happen. They are a serious business that loves to have fun. One of their core values is humor.

For more information you can give them a ring at 800-523-3958 or visit their website at www.techgroupinc.com. They are located at 244 West Main, Spokane, WA 99207.

~*~

Travel Max / Maxim

Travel Max provides travel assignments to RNs, OR techs and therapists. Their local Maxim offices provide contracts to all healthcare positions. They cover all 50 states for travel, but do not currently do international assignments. The time from acceptance of application to first day on the job for those nurses ready to go can vary, depending on the client's request and the speed that a nurse turns in their paperwork. Most range from five days to three weeks. They are a part of Maxim Healthcare, which gives them access to a lot of needs. Their division is medium in size and they do things to make sure that each nurse is treated like gold. They have dedicated consultants that remain with a nurse on all assignments, and they have direct phone access to their assigned consultant.

Personal service is what drives their operations. No matter what questions a nurse has, they can contact their consultant and they will find the answer for them. Through Maxim you also have local contacts where they have an assignment that makes the travel experience better. They have internal workers on call for that very reason. Answering services cannot make decisions. Their on-call person knows the business and can assist with emergencies immediately.

They offer a full package of benefits, including insurance, 401K, bonuses, private housing and top pay. They tailor make their package to the need of the traveler, along with extensive professional insurance.

Their focus on personal attention sets them apart. They constantly strive to shape their operation to make the travel experience unmatched. This is reflected also in their unique advantage of a local contact while you are on your assignment. Their commitment is to provide the best service to their hospitals and their nurses. They are very straightforward with their staff and place a lot of value on building a trusting relationship.

For more information they can be found at 3550 Buschwood Park Drive, Suite 230, Tampa, FL 33618. Their phone is listed as 888-800-1855, and their website can be found at www.travelmax.com.

~*~

Travel Nurse Across America

Travel Nurse across America (TNAA) is a company where service begins day one. Their company slogan, "Exceeding Expectations," is a complete representation of their dedication to travelers' needs by providing personal attention, commitment and support throughout every assignment. Because TNAA is a medium-sized agency, they are able to offer access to jobs that smaller staffing companies can't, without sacrificing personal attention and customer service travelers deserve and expect. The company strives to create a fulfilling, pleasant and trouble-free "no surprises" process to help health care professionals explore the country.

TNAA specializes in thirteen-week assignments with opportunities for multiple extensions. Typically, the application process takes two to four weeks from start to finish, but depending on the hospital's and nurse's needs, assignments can be "fast tracked" and processed in a matter of days. Recruiting Specialists, Quality Assurance Assignment Specialists and an on-site on-staff Director of Nursing and Clinical Nurse Liaison are available and on standby 24/7 to offer any help along the way.

"Your Way is Paid" is a recent program in which TNAA absorbs all costs associated with building a traveler's file in preparation for a secured assignment. This includes medical expenses, (i.e. titers, drug screens, physicals), state licensure, credentials, continuing education, competency testing, and a generous travel reimbursement program that involves no receipts, reducing the stress travelers may feel as they embark on their journeys, as well as streamlining the process to help travelers get on assignment faster.

TNAA offers some of the most outstanding benefits in the industry with insurance, 401K with company match, and a loyalty points program all beginning the first day worked. Their health insurance has different levels of coverage, including free insurance, which gives travelers medical coverage options to meet their specific needs. They also offer professional liability insurance at no charge, a vision plan, short term and long-term disability, and life insurance. In addition to these coverages, TNAA also offers a Tax-Advantage program for qualified travelers that maximizes their take-home pay, as well as extra income that is available through completion, extension, referral, and hospital bonuses.

TNAA fully recognizes that health care professionals can choose from a number of agencies that offer standard perks like free private housing, free utilities, free insurance, etc. TNAA cultivates relationships with travelers because they know it's the people who are important and who ensure longevity in any business. The company has earned countless loyal travelers who attest to TNAA's personal service and often leave comments on the testimonial portion of their website: www.nurse.tv.

They accept applicants of all specialties and experiences as long as they are licensed for work in the US. If an applicant is not quite ready to travel, they are happy to provide resources to help gain the experience and knowledge needed for the applicant's future assignments.

Travel Nurse across America can be reached at 11300 Cantrell Road, Suite 102, Little Rock, AR 72212 and phoned at 800-240-2526.

~*~

Travel Nurse Network

Travel Nurse Network (TNN) offers luxury housing that is located near the facility and carefully researched to insure the traveler's safety. The housing is free, private, furnished, with utilities included. Housing packages are customized for the travelers' needs, with options for housing packages. Monthly stipends are also available, equaling the value of the housing offered in the area. That would be a monthly non-taxed check.

TNN is a family-owned business, originating in Florida. The family relocated to Chicago, IL, expanding and adding a local per diem division. Travelers should be assured when they call the office, as anyone they speak to should be able to assist them in their travel needs. Members of the original family still work in the office. Phone calls will always be returned, even after business hours, to accommodate the needs of shift working nurses and therapists.

They offer tax advantages, which enables a portion of each pay to be exempt from taxes. Hourly rates are very competitive and are customized to reflect the traveler's needs. The best bonus is their PPO, top-of-the-line premium medical insurance.

Travel Nurse Network is a specialized company that employs nursing professionals to serve nursing professionals. TNN's recruiters are nurses with recent healthcare experience. They are able to collect the correct information to clearly represent the current nursing positions and to match nurses based on their specialty, skills level, and travel needs. You are part of a family when you work for TNN. They welcome your families to join you on location. They enjoy the pictures and stories their nurses share with them. To show their loyalty to you, TNN offers one-week paid vacation on your one-year anniversary with the company. TNN wants you to further your nursing career while enjoying it.

For more information on Travel Nurse Network you can contact them at 300 W. Adams Street, Suite 326, Chicago, IL 60606. You may also call them at 800.510.8802 or visit their website at www.travelnursenetwork.com.

~*~

Trinity Healthcare Staffing Group

"I couldn't find a staffing company that kept its promises. So I started one," Matt Floyd, R.N, Founder, President, and CEO says.

As a former traveling critical care nurse, Matt had become all too familiar with the infuriating drill: Showing up to bewildered looks instead of secured housing; paychecks that rarely landed in his hands on time, and when they did, were routinely for reduced or inaccurate amounts; and perhaps worst of all, there was never anywhere or anyone to turn to to seek counsel from or just sympathize with him.

Trinity Healthcare was born out of that frustration. Matt founded the company in 1999 around a very simple idea: *Doing what we say we'll do.* That translates into offering medical facilities higher quality healthcare professionals, and offering healthcare professionals a company that keeps its promises. It's made them one of the fastest growing and most trusted staffing agencies in the country, and it's why you'll find a home at Trinity too.

Trinity Healthcare Staffing Group offers travel, per diem, and temp-to-perm placement for nursing and allied healthcare professionals. Trinity is a national company offering travel assignments all across the country, with per diem staffing available through their branch offices.

In 2004 Trinity was named on the Inc. 500 list for being one of the fastest growing privately owned companies in the country, as well as being recognized as one of the fastest growing companies in South Carolina in 2003 and 2004.

Trinity has also been awarded the Joint Commission's Gold Seal of Approval. Trinity offers the following benefits to their travel nurses: major medical, dental, vision, prescription drug coverage along with life insurance of $25,000, workman's compensation, general liability insurance, professional liability insurance, 401K, completion bonuses for quite a few assignments, and an unlimited general referral bonus. You receive all of this, in addition to one of the highest pay packages in the industry. While their employees are covered by Trinity, they are rather conservative and of the belief that one can never have too much professional liability insurance. So give us a call and let us help you help others, like the unique specialists you are.

For more information, contact them at 1834 Sally Hill Farms Blvd., P.O. Box 5955, Florence, SC 29501, 877-417-9507, www.TrinityHSG.com.

~*~

Trustaff

Trustaff offers travel contracts ranging in length from 8 weeks to one year for Registered Nurses. They also staff Pharmacists, Registered Nurses and Allied Health Professionals for permanent positions. In some areas they also offer per diem/PRN shifts. They currently staff all 50 states, as well as the American Virgin Islands. Nurses can be on assignment within one week after all paperwork is turned in and the assignment is accepted.

They are a middle-sized company that is quickly moving into the large business division. You can expect top-of-the-line personal service with their company. They offer real 24/7 contact for all of their health care professionals, not just an answering service. You will speak with someone who can get things done, whatever that might be.

Trustaff offers tax advantage and all-inclusive pay plans—health, dental, and vision coverage through United Healthcare with Nurse's Choice between three plans including a 90/10 plan, free life insurance, referral bonuses up to $1500, sign-on bonuses, completion bonuses, extension bonuses, loyalty bonuses, paid time-off with each assignment, 24/7 support for all of their travelers, customizable benefit packages, weekly direct deposit with online viewing, licensure assistance and reimbursement. I believe their professional insurance is very good, but extra insurance is just that—added insurance, and that is never bad.

They pride themselves on offering all the benefits, great pay and locations that the biggest companies do, while still maintaining the support and service of a smaller company. They also offer some of the highest pay rates in the industry, featuring several pay and benefit packages for their healthcare professionals to choose from. They thank all of their healthcare professionals for their continuing service to their communities, families and friends.

Trustaff can be contacted at 4270 Glendale-Milford Rd, Cincinnati, OH 45242 or called at 877-880-0346. Their website is located at www.trustaff.com.

~*~

Worldwide Travel Staffing

WTS offers 13-week travel nursing assignments in all specialties. Other durations are also available. They cover all areas of the United States and can have you placed in as little as seven days. They also place nurses in the UAE, Australia, New Zealand, London, and Ireland. They are R.N. owned and operated and they understand the nuances of travel nursing.

Their company is rapidly growing, but it is doing so from a small starting point. It is the friendly customer service that is causing nurses to refer their friends. Their 24-hour phone service is always available for staff.

Traditional Blue Cross/Blue Shield is available on the first day of your first assignment. Generous tax advantage plans are available. They will individually tailor their compensation to suit specific needs. They offer a retirement vesting account with 3% company match with "Free Money." Free private housing is available, as is full travel reimbursements,; $1,000 to $5,000 completion bonuses are standard; other benefits include up to $2,000 referral bonuses, weekly paychecks, and weekly meals and lodging allowances. Nurses have the option of a quality health insurance plan. You will not find better medical insurance coverage in the entire travel nurse industry.

They are different from the other companies in that the owner is not only a registered nurse, but a master's prepared psychiatric nurse. Call and find out why they are the most caring company at 866-633-3700. You can find them at 2829 Sheridan Drive, Tonawanda, NY 14150. Their website can be found at www.WorldwideTravelStaffing.com.

~*~

Valley Healthcare Systems

Valley Healthcare Systems specialize in travel nurse assignments nationwide, as well as local per diem/registry. They can have you placed within four days for a travel assignment and two days for per diem / registry.

They have 325 nurses, and each of their nurses are treated as though they were their only nurse, and they have a night nurse on call 24 hours per day and reachable via phone. You will never get an answering service.

Benefits include paid medical benefits, 401K, direct deposit, weekly paychecks, fully furnished private housing/ housing allowance, airfare to and from your assignment or a travel allowance and a rental car. They provide top-notch professional and general liability insurance that is A+ rated.

They pay higher than their competitors and still offer a personal touch from start to finish. Their nurses stay with them, and I do mean stay with them! Their average length of tenure is close to four continuous contracts.

For more information they can be contacted at Valley Healthcare Systems Inc 11290 Pyrites Way Suite 200A, Gold River, CA 95670. Their phone number is 800-953-0508, and their website can be found at www.vhcsystems.com.

~*~

Valley Medical Staffing

Valley Medical Staffing offers 13 to 26-week travel nursing assignments. Occasionally they will have 4 to 8 week opportunities, but those are rare. They specialize in California assignments, but have branched out into other states including Washington, Oregon, Colorado and Alaska. They can have you on the road in as little as four days, but it just depends if all the pieces of the puzzle fall into place. They staff mainly RN's, but they do occasionally have LVN and Radiology Tech positions available.

They are a small travel nurse company and you definitely will not be a number. The lead staffing specialist is a former traveler herself. She will treat you the way she expected to be treated as a traveler.

Hopefully problems can be solved during the daytime hours, but she always keeps her phone with her. She gives all of her travelers her personal cell phone number so she can be reached whenever necessary, so the answer to the question is "Yes, they do take care of problems at night."

They provide weekly direct deposit. You will be paid the Friday after your first week's work, corporate-style housing or housing stipend, medical insurance provided at no cost to the traveler, subsidy for family members, a 401K plan is available, and travel pay. They also provide adequate professional insurance.

Their greatest asset is their fairness and honesty. They will not submit you without your expressed permission. They are independently owned and not looking to sell. The owners have decided to have a former travel nurse as their lead recruiter so the nurses might feel more cared for themselves. You will be appreciated!

For more information contact them at 3685 Mt. Diablo Blvd Ste. 351 Lafayette , CA 94549 , or phone them at 1-888-267-4174. Their website can be found at www.vmstaffing.com.

~*~

Wesley Medical Staffing

Wesley Medical Staffing offers per diem, short term, long term, and temp-to-perm opportunities for RN's, LPN's, and CNA's nationwide. They can do hospital, office, long-term acute care, and correctional assignments throughout the United States, including Hawaii and Alaska.

They are a very small company with offices positioned strategically to specifically target the high traffic areas where travel nurses want to go. Their average placement time after acceptance is generally dependent on the client facility. Most facilities for travel assignments allow the nurse to start ASAP (or as soon as they can get there). Typical turn around time after acceptance is about a week to ten days. They work very hard to make sure that they completely understand the needs and goals of their nurses to give them their "best fit" in assignments.

They have someone on their phones twenty-four/seven to answer any questions or address any concerns that their nurses may have. If there is a clinical concern or patient care issue, their nurse directors are also available to discuss issues on a one-on-one basis.

Wesley Medical provides generous sign-on and referral bonuses, paid private housing (or stipends), paid travel (or stipends), education reimbursement, and health care reimbursement. They believe that their company's insurance carrier is very thorough and comprehensive, but as a nurse the owner has always carried her own professional liability insurance and makes this same recommendation to all nurses working for their company.

Their personal service is what sets Wesley apart from other companies. They truly care about their nurses and it shows in their bookings and in their retention numbers. They would love for all travel nurses to take a look at Wesley and give them a try. They are not the biggest and flashiest company out there, but their *people know* healthcare and nursing and they would love to help you find your next assignment.

For more information about Wesley Medical Staffing you can phone them at 866-295-9306 or visit their website at www.wesleymedicalstaffing.com. Their offices are located at 801 E. Morehead St., Suite 305, Charlotte, NC 28202.

LaRue Tradition That Shall Not Be Broken...

"Love At First Type"
Published January 2001

"Crazy Thoughts Of Passion"
Published January 2003

"Highway Hypodermics: Your Road To Travel Nursing"
Published January 2005

"Highway Hypodermics: Travel Nursing 2007"
Published January 2007

"Crazy Thoughts Of An Online Romance"
Published January 2008

"Highway Hypodermics: On The Road Again"
Published January 2009

"Highway Hypodermics: Travel Nursing 2011"
Scheduled To Be Published January 2011

Love At First Type:
An Online Romance Based On A True Story

Paperback: 156 pages
Publisher: Booksurge Publishing (January, 2001)
Out Of Print

Nurse Kathy's life was changed when she met Jack over the internet. They are not only separated by 1000 miles, but also 24 years! They find themselves chatting more and more each day. Soon they begin to contemplate the idea of making their romance a reality. The odds are against them...

Can they make an Internet Romance an everlasting Reality Romance? Is it worth going against all those odds? Is there really such a thing as *Love At First Type?*

~*~

"*Love At First Type* is a story that tugs at your heart strings and makes you a true believer of romance - and that soul mates will find each other no matter what. I could not put this book down. I had to keep reading to see what happened next to "Sassy" and "Repairmen." I highly recommend it to anyone who has ever thought about having an online relationship." *Kristie Leigh Maguire, author of award winning romance novels, "Desert Heat", and "Cabin Fever"*

"...LaRue spins a tale that will capture the reader in the first sentence and will keep them spell bound til the end." *Kim Roberts, author of "Everlasting" and "A Chance Worth Taking."*

"... LaRue is a promising new talent."
Brenda Bailey, Literary Agent

Crazy Thoughts Of Passion

Paperback: 98 pages
Publisher: Booksurge Publishing (January, 2003)
Out Of Print

Kaitlyn Malloy is a registered nurse with her hands full at Madison Acute Geriatric-Psychiatric Hospital. The newly admitted Gladys Rosanthol had been brought into the hospital with an acute maniac episode. Kaitlyn had no other choice but to give her an anti-anxiety medication.

Lance Rosanthol was stupefied when he saw his mother. She wasn't just relaxed; she was comatose! He is taking his mother out of that crazy hospital, and he doesn't care what that Nurse Malloy says!

Kaitlyn certainly didn't need anyone questioning her nursing capabilities! But why did crazy thoughts of passion keep entering her mind every time that she looked at Mrs. Rosanthol's handsome son? Naturally, nursing ethics complicates this situation. She definitely doesn't need him to complicate her life!

~*~

...A short book, Crazy Thoughts of Passion is big on characters and ideas, it's almost as if you are facing the dilemmas with Kaitlyn and wondering what you would do in that same situation. An easy read, the book's pages seem to turn themselves. ...A must for any romance fan. *Reviewed by Annette Gisby, author of "Silent Screams" and "Shadows of the Rose."*

...Ms. LaRue's own experience as a nurse lends an aura of realism to this poignant romance. You will fall in love right along with these two wonderful people who must first deal with modern life before they can indulge their "Crazy Thoughts of Passion." *Reviewed by Kathleen Walls, Author of Last Step and Georgia's Ghostly Getaways*

Highway Hypodermics: Your Road Map To Travel Nursing

Paperback: 156 pages
Publisher: Star Publish (January, 2005)
www.starpublishllc.com
ISBN: 1932993169

Highway Hypodermic by Epstein LaRue may be a one-of-a-kind book. That is a rarity but apparently true. After a search on Amazon and a couple of other online bookstores, I found nothing currently in print on the subject of making nursing-on-wheels a career.

LaRue says she wrote this book so that a professional nurse "can make an informed decision about your career change into travel nursing." But Highway Hypodermics will also be valuable for anyone considering a nursing career of any kind for Larue doesn't mince words. She tells all she knows about the distractions, difficulties and benefits of becoming any kind of a nurse as well as fully informing readers about a nursing niche that few others could tell them about.

LaRue's strength is twofold. She speaks from experience—lots of it—and she speaks in a casual, straight-from-the-heart voice. Her honesty is impeccable. My favorite chapters are those in which she reveals her own journals. By doing so, she opens a window on her world—both personal and in terms of her chosen career. We often look to memoir to learn more about ourselves; perhaps all those considering nursing will find it an advantage to do that before they choose this difficult but rewarding field. By combining this mirror to her life in a how-to book, LaRue offers up a nursing guide like no other.

Reviewed by Carolyn Howard-Johnson is the award-winning author of This is the Place and Harkening: A Collection of Stories Remembered. The Frugal Book Promoter: How to Do What Your Publisher Won't was just named USA Book News "Best Books of 2004." Award. Learn more at http://carolynhowardjohnson.com/ Contact Reviewer: HoJoNews@aol.com

Highway Hypodermics: Travel Nursing 2007

Paperback: 372 pages
Publisher: Star Publish (January, 2007)
ISBN: 1932883657

Whether snow skiing in Idaho, viewing the sunset from helicopter pad on the top of a hospital in Arizona, gazing at covered bridges in Vermont, or taking a long walk on the beach in Florida, travel nursing is an excellent way to get paid while exploring the United States. Although Highway Hypodermics: Your Road Map To Travel Nursing was written in 2005 with some great information about travel nursing, the next edition, Highway Hypodermics: Travel Nursing 2007, brings expanded knowledge about the field of travel nursing. Not only do you get the basics of travel nursing, but additional information is provided on the rewards and drawbacks of travel nursing and making the decision to travel, expanded knowledge on what travel companies are all about and how to choose the right one, all about JCAHO certification, which destinations are the best and how to choose a destination, information on traveling in a recreational vehicle, home-schooling your child while on the road, and additional information on licensing requirements, not to mention all you would ever need to know about travel nursing and your taxes.

Crazy Thoughts Of An Online Romance

Paperback: 320 pages
Publisher: Star Publish (January, 2008)
ISBN: 1932993851

A fictional nursing duet: Crazy Thoughts of Passion (originally published in 2003) and Love At First Type: On Online Romance, Based On A True Story (originally published in 2001) with the added NEVER RELEASED Epstein's Guide To Online Romance. In Book One, Nurse Kathy's life was changed when she met Jack over the internet. They are not only separated by 1000 miles, but also 24 years! They find themselves chatting more and more each day. Soon they begin to contemplate the idea of making their romance a reality. The odds are against them... Can they make an Internet Romance an everlasting Reality Romance? Is it worth going against all those odds? Is there really such a thing as Love At First Type? In Book Two, Kaitlyn Malloy is a registered nurse with her hands full at Madison Acute Geriatric-Psychiatric Hospital. Lance Rosanthol has a mother who is having anxiety attacks, but the real panic starts when sparks ignite a passionate fire between Lance and Kaitlyn. Naturally, nursing ethics complicates this situation. An intriguing look at nursing, ethics, romance, and. Crazy Thoughts Of Passion.

Got Nurses?

Understanding The Traveling Nurse In Effort To Retain Nurses

The travel nursing industry is growing at an extremely accelerated rate in the last five years. Once there were only a handful of staffing companies, today there are over 200 companies that specialize in travel nursing. The task of finding out what nurses want and supplying their needs has become an ever so daunting.

Recruiting nurses to join your organization is tough enough without adding the chore of retaining the nurses once you have got them on your team. With a little understanding of what nurses what, how to read their personalities, and how to treat them, you're job just got a little easier.

"Got Nurses" is a one hour program developed by Epstein LaRue as a tool to give travel companies a peak into the world of travel nursing from the other side.

~*~

"As new employees to the travel industry, we thoroughly enjoyed reading Highway Hypodermics: Your Road Map to Travel Nursing and listening to the program, "Got Nurses?" Epi gives a better understanding to what a healthcare traveler is looking for which is a necessity for any good recruiter. She captures the adventures and advantages of Healthcare Traveling from a traveling nurse's perspective. The "Got Nurses" program combined with the "Highway Hypodermic" book series has astronomical value to a travel nursing company!"

Trinity Healthcare Staffing Group – Recruitment Team

~*~

For more information about this one hour inservice contact Epstein at: highwayhypo@yaho.com

Websites of Interest:

www.highwayhypodermics.com
Epstein's travel nursing homepage where you will find up-to-date information about travel nursing companies, hospitals, and more stories from traveling nurses.

www.epsteinlarue.com
Epstein LaRue's author homepage full of valuable information about her books, medical consulting for writer's, and tips on how for you to get started in a profitable writing career.

www.travelnursinghighway.blogspot.com
Travel nursing blog where Traveling nurses can come together and discuss the everyday adventures of travel nursing and find out more information.

www.myspace.com/nurse_epi
Epstein's MySpace page

groups.myspace.com/TravelNursingAlliance
health.groups.yahoo.com/group/highwayhypodermics/
Epstein's MySpace and Yahoo groups from which her eZine announcements are made.

forums.delphiforums.com/travelnurses/
A community of past, present, and future traveling nurses who support each other in an amazing forum.

www.ultimatenurse.com
Another great website forum for traveling nurses with company and hospital reviews also.

www.pantravelers.org
The Professional Association of Nurse Travelers a non-profit organization, exists to serve the interests of all healthcare travelers.

Who Is Epstein LaRue?

The writing world calls her Epstein LaRue, but reality calls her "Kay." No matter what you know her by, she is a lady of many talents. She has been a nurse since 1992, and has worked on medical, surgical, emergency, telemetry, rehabilitation, and psychiatric units.

In January 2001, Epstein's first book, "Love At First Type: An Online Romance Based On A True Story," was published. This fictional novel is about how she and her husband met online. This book was recently requested by an independent filmmaker for possible production in the near future.

In January 2003 her second book, "Crazy Thoughts Of Passion" was released. It is a fictional medical romance about a nurse who falls in love with a patient's son.

In January 2005 her third and most successful book, "Highway Hypodermics: Your Road Map To Travel Nursing" was published. Although only on the road for two years, everything that she learned in those two years was put into the book. In September of 2005, this book was recognized by USA Book News as one of the top finalist for professional book of the year.

In January 2007 (can you see the trend yet....) "Highway Hypodermics: Travel Nursing 2007" was released by Star Publish (www.starpublishllc.com). This book soared up the charts on Amazon and made it to Number One three times in the Nursing, Trends, Issues and Roles category.

In January 2008, Epstein put together her first two novels, "Love At First Type" and "Crazy Thoughts Of Passion" together with her new publisher in "Crazy Thoughts Of An Online Romance."

Other recent accomplishments include having her article, "Top 10 Reasons To Love Travel Nursing" published in one of nursing's most prestigious magazines, Nursing2004. She was also named as a Traveler of the Year by Healthcare Traveler magazine in December 2005, and in 2008 she had three articles published by "ORNursing2008."

LaRue keeps herself busy during the month by publishing a monthly eZine about travel nursing, "Highway Happenings" and leading a group of authors who do things "Not The Usual Way" commonly referred as the NUW Author Community (http://groups.yahoo.com/group/NUW/).

Travel nursing is a dream that has become a reality. She currently spends her summer at her home office in Idaho freelance writing and working per-diem, and continues to travel south in winter with her husband. Step into her world and shoot yourself down the road with Highway Hypodermics.